The Kaleb Sutra

7

day

SEX

detox

Front Cover design by MJ.
Crash tested on MJ & CJ (Thanks!)

International Standard Book Number (ISBN): 978-83-7946-021-2

www.kalebsutra.com

Disclaimer.

The 7 Day Sex Detox does not take your individual dietary needs and/or pre-existing medical conditions into account. This detox is designed for educational purposes and not intended as a substitute for professional medical advice. Always consult your doctor with questions/concerns you may have about your health. Do not disregard professional medical advice or prior knowledge you may have toward your own individual medical conditions where applicable over the information contained in this detox. The Kaleb Sutra has adapted this lifestyle detox to guide you towards achieving better sexual fitness, and has made every effort to provide safe and practical advice, however waives liability to the extent permissible by law.

A QUICK NOTE

The 7 Day Sex Detox has been prepared with all readers in mind. It doesn't matter whether you're in your sexual prime, or pushing fifty and beyond (and everywhere in between). This detox won't judge you on your fitness levels, whether you're fit or out of shape – this one's for you. Guys and girls are welcome and whether you're into guys or girls (or both) you're invited to come and take the 7-day challenge too! Anyone from any walk of life (or even any culture that may imply that sex isn't up for discussion) should keep reading – as every one of us who has picked up these pages shares one common goal: The desire to step up our sex lives (whatever that may involve) and become a better playmate. And in our own personal journeys of sexuality – sexual discovery and sexual fulfillment, the most important thing to remember is that it's never too late to take a leap of faith and improve ourselves for the better, even if there is no one who's watching!

PS.

Whether you' re a 9 to 5 or more of a or graveyard shift type, breakfast or meal one can be taken at whatever time of day you usually go for it, same goes for lunch or meal two and so on. Take the same approach to the AMs and PMs referenced in this detox. Mornings/afternoons/evenings are basically the beginning/ middle/end parts of each day. For those of you with mornings starting when everyone else's evenings are in full swing – you know the drill, switch it up so that you're starting on the detoxing whatever time of the day it is that YOU are having that first meal!

This Detox is broken down into 7 days. Each day includes a breakdown of daily goals, energy levels, meal plans, recipes and ingredients, together with a downloadable and printable resource kit with shopping lists and quick reference guides to all of the do's and don'ts designed to help make the 7 days as easy as possible to wrap your head around! Be sure to visit *kalebsutra.com* for all the latest.

INTRODUCTION - *PLAYMATE 'A'*

THINK BACK to the last time you thought to yourself, *I am so not going down on you tonight.* Or picture that last time when you were in the final seconds of the most intense, mind-blowing oral sex (as is usually the case, in that whole heat of the moment thing). Then just as you're about to release every bit of all that tension, an unwilling set of lips suddenly pulls away, in preference of letting you drown in your own sorrows, over the thought of having to go near even the slightest drop. (Notwithstanding the off chance that you might get a taste of your own medicine, in the hope that you will then have some idea of how nasty you have let that part of sex actually taste).

Hate Cum? You're not alone. But we're not just talking about that here. Let's create a mental picture of what's involved in the overall *scent structure* of each of us. This can be summed up as *body odors* in a broad sense and likened to both taste and smell, two of the key senses involved in any sexual experience. And to keep it simple, let's summarize *taste*, *smell* and *scent structure* into one logical thought process that can be used going forward: *scent*.

So, your scent can include everything from ejaculation (whether you're a guy or girl – remember back to that big 'O' you were having earlier?) (And I'm just going to call it cum, ok! Who, besides high school teachers uses the word 'ejaculation' anyway?!), pre-cum and that moist state girls get into when they're a little hot under the collar - through to sweat and urine. (Urine is such a clinical term I know, but I can't help but associate the word 'piss' with some vague level of political incorrectness, despite sounding far more sexually adhesive But let's just keep it clinical for the sake of said *'PC'* being some sort of moral glue that I hope will keep the all-round controversial subject matter of this whole story above board). And my final word on all of this 'loaded vocabulary' before someone beats me to the punch is pretty straightforward. The more than likely reason for which you've picked up this book is to try to address something in the ballpark of your sexual scent being a little bit off key, *or* you're trying to take some positive steps toward improving your sexual identity as a whole. For that reason you're (hopefully) not too straight-laced (ok, sensitive!) toward the general subject matter. Which if in reality you are, you probably shouldn't be reading this book anyway. Despite the fact that this book contains very little about sex itself - it's more of a 'how-to' guide to understanding what's involved in the behind-the-scenes personal prep-work toward achieving greater sexual fulfillment and being a better playmate. So if you were in fact counting on something a little more sexually fulfilling (albeit the fact that what's contained in this little book is ultimately *aimed* at achieving just that - have we all forgotten about delayed gratification this early in the game?) you should likely be flipping through the pages that came *before* these ones.

Playmate – *as simple as it sounds, your sexual partner.*

Ok, so it's time for the reality check of reality checks. More often than not, your sexual scent will *err* on the side of being unpleasant. And when it comes to sex, the big 'O' and everything in between, ~~tasting like crap~~ playing on the 'offensive' just isn't sexy. Unfortunately, this is the part where political correctness just creeps its ugly way into the equation again (always knowing when to make a potentially good moment awkward). And combined with some good old fashioned bad (or complete lack thereof) communication skills; sex can quite innocently become prohibitive, less engaging and/or just plain not happening. It seems hard to point the finger at either playmate without pointing the finger at both. Is it playmate A's fault (for having a bad scent in whatever activity was concerned) or playmate B's fault, for not saying anything about it straight up? (and in doing so, not creating positive open channels of communication, which is essential to any healthy relationship, be that sexual in nature or otherwise) As in the case of playmate B - not saying anything about it, and resorting to sexual avoidance or closed mindedness (and rightfully so, I mean would *YOU* go down on that?) is the unfortunate reality of what happens between playmates.

6

Take this example of a simple Internet search on *my boyfriend smells when I'm trying to go down...* or *why does my girlfriend's.. smell like...* (you get the idea) which will provide hours of trawling through countless forums on the subject, and it doesn't end there I'm afraid. Upon (not even really extensive) browsing, you can find the terms 'boyfriend' and 'girlfriend' become replaced with more permanent fixtures, such as 'husband' and 'wife', which perhaps is the most disconcerting of all. The fact that sexual miscommunication can allow for what could otherwise be a potentially long, healthy and enjoyable sex life, lead to years of dysfunction – *vis-a-vis* trawling through the internet for answers to what to do to avoid 'that experience' really does leave a lot to think about. If only more of us just had the guts to say outright, *'babe, you taste like crap'*.

So back to playmate B - that's a problem, which probably can't be resolved as easily as it sounds, (without launching into a theological debate on human nature – which is *clearly* far from happening at this point) but this little set of self-helping pages is not actually about playmate B (unless you *are* playmate B buying this book to give to playmate A in the first place). It's about playmate A stepping up to the plate and becoming a *responsible playmate*. Taking the small steps needed to improve on 'A's sexual scent can go a long way, and it all starts with asking the question – *why does my cum taste like crap?* Now this question wasn't intended to tackle the world head on, and make everyone love the stuff. Sex *is* an individual *taste* and the reality is that some people hate the stuff and never will consider going anywhere near it. What we're trying to do here in fact is turn the bad around into something a bit more *sugar coated*, and in doing so make it less of a bitter pill to swallow - for those of us who enjoy enough versatility in our sex lives, to appreciate every bit of it. That wasn't a rhetorical question either, just by the way. It's not one of those *'why do I have to go to work today'* moments, not by a long shot. It has everything to do with taking a look at the reality of *'well if you didn't get plastered again last night'* life wouldn't seem like such a chore the morning after – and point blank, you wouldn't taste like *crap* either. Did you really think all that whiskey was doing you any favors? So in effect – both *late for work* and *no quickie* that morning, is probably going to make for an all round *crap day* – yep that's looking, feeling *and* tasting like it. Get the picture yet?

So if what playmate A does is make those small changes needed to improve on the scent that was so unpleasant in the first place, then playmate B wouldn't be put in the position of having to spend hours late at night on the internet, trying to do A's job for them, would they? *(or having to make 'A' sleep on the couch, when stumbling home that night, all 'A' was busy thinking of was that juicy set of lips waiting at home, ready to go down…)* The reality? Well yep, that second bit is clearly not happening and as for the rest - there's plenty of other *positions* that 'B' would rather be spending hours late at night having to worry about.

Sexual Responsibility: *Maintaining a positive sexual fitness in order to provide a positive sexual experience for you and your playmate.*

And whether you're 'A' or 'B' or *both* (versatility is after all key to a healthy sex life) then there's one simple idea, which may in fact help to solve some of your problems: sex detox.

And let's face it - we could all do with a great tasting playmate 'A' any day, couldn't we?

A discussion on sexual fitness would not be complete without drawing our attention to the other real issue concerned when any sexual endeavor is concerned - performance. So eating healthy, living well - *what does it all have to do with your sexual fitness anyway?* Short answer – more than you may think. *It's only just sex though, right?* True, but start by taking a more organic approach and think about sex for what it actually involves – physical fitness. And like any athlete or 'Sunday afternoon shooting a few hoops with the boys' type, in order to achieve a peak level of performance (or just the ability to not make a complete *dumbass* of yourself in front of your mates) there's a few basic things you need to pay attention to. Mental alertness, stamina, endurance, *et-F-c.* - that part we all know. What in most cases we don't lend enough thought to however is that sex is a physical activity – and a challenging one at that. A great sex life involves a high level of sexual fitness in order to explore how to maximize its full potential, whilst enjoying every part of the process. I think by this point as a society we will have embraced the age old concept of *we are what we eat* a hundred times over. And that's no joke - particularly when it comes to your sexual fitness. What you get out of your body is only ever going to be as good as what you put in. So taking a step back to figure out what that actually means is a good place to start.

Sexual Fitness: *Your sexual fitness ultimately relates to your willingness and ability toward doing the deed, both on a cognitive and physical level (likening it to 'sexual energy' per say, wouldn't be too far off the mark either).*

Let's dive in little further: your cognitive ability and willingness to have sex relates to your mood, state of mind, sexual drive and general interest toward having anything to do with it. Your physical ability and willingness to have sex on the other hand can be split two ways. The first of these relates directly to your ability to *fire up those engines*. In the case of guys it means *getting it up* - girls on the other hand would liken that process to *getting those juices flowing*. But the commonality between both guys and girls toward this part of sexual fitness is the reality that our bodies are largely similar in what actually makes us tick. Let's use watermelons and pomegranates to highlight the basics. Watermelon is a great staple fruit towards conditioning a positive level of sexual fitness. One of the benefits of watermelon is the increased flow of oxygen in your bloodstream (due to the high levels of citrulline it contains). Which in the case of us guys will indeed help to *get it up* and as for you girls, increased blood flow during sexual activity will heighten the experience and stimulate those places that count the most – giving one of the elements of sexual fitness a big thumbs up. Try pomegranate too – both guys and girls that drink pomegranate juice regularly, have been found to experience increased levels of testosterone, which boosts the sexual fitness of all concerned. So it's really a case of *same, same but different* in it's truest form. What makes us tick, however similar is very different in nature, but the 'how-to guide' for conditioning our sexual fitness is going to look much the same for all playmates, independent of what we're packing down there.

The second part of your physical ability and willingness to have sex is as simple as the concept suggests - it describes the relationship between a playmate's physical strength and endurance toward sexual activity. This detox is going to cover both cognitive and physical elements of your sexual fitness, but physical strength and endurance (the second part of the physical role of sexual fitness) is going to be the focus of WOOD WORK, the follow up to BANANA SMOOTHIES, which will be available as the next set of pages, following these.

Lifestyle factors play a big role in determining your sexual fitness. We already know that what you put into your body will more or less determine what you're going to be getting out of it later. So that seems to make all the more sense with the eating healthy part of the equation. Much like your sexual scent, your sexual energy on every level is an important part of your sexual fitness. And the key to achieving a harmonious (perfect world, I know) sexual balance is recognizing that both these two elements are so closely interrelated with doing and having *the big 'O', Over and Over* again.

So what have we managed to string together? That eating *crap* not only makes you taste and smell that way, but it's also not going to be doing you any favors when it comes to actually doing the deed either. Limiting BLACK LIST food from your diet and balancing the intake of RED LIST with BLUE, YELLOW and GREEN LISTS foods will do more than you think to help boost your sexual fitness in both the short and long term (so there is some instant gratification in there somewhere after all - thankfully). And of course both those lists are found (somewhere) on the following pages. To paint (another) straightforward picture, have a think about basic physical abilities of the fit vs. the unfit. Those of us who have managed to pay attention to a lifestyle balanced with fitness and a reasonable diet are generally a lot more active and interested in physical activity in general - to which I relate sexual fitness and a general willingness to explore your sexuality, directly. Less thought through lifestyle choices on the other hand will generally relate to the opposite taking place where your sexual fitness is concerned, which will basically make you less prone to getting out and actually enjoying life, and yep - sex.

The winning thing about life nevertheless is that it is never too late to get your ass into gear and embrace everything there is to do toward making a change for the better and taking on board more positive lifestyle choices - to improve your cognitive, physical and sexual abilities across the board. For that very simple and forgiving reason, I invite you to join me on this seven day detox. Yep, it's all about sharing the challenges and personal milestones as we know, but as far as challenges go - seven days is not a large whack out of your life - and really, it's only the first three or four that you're heavily reducing your food intake to get that whole greater good sort of stuff happening. So giving your body a spring break may be just the thing you need to find and achieve that little bit more sexual fitness and fulfillment. And worst case – well you've taken a moment or two to think twice about what you're actually doing to your body and maybe even picked up a thing or two along the way – so not all bad, in the greater scheme of things.

BLACK LIST

Foods to Avoid

As the name suggests, this list contains a basic list of foods that are not going to do you any favors in terms of your sexual fitness - contributing less favorably to various aspects. So the best thing you can do is to keep them to a minimum and as far as foods are concerned, find other foods to replace them with. These lists are provided as starting guides and are designed to point you in the right direction. Once you have a feel for what each of them covers, you should explore each of the lists further and use your own experiences and trial and error to develop your lists further and determine which foods work for you and which ones don't.

- CAULIFLOWER
- BROCCOLI
- ASPARAGUS
- CABBAGE
- SPINACH
- POTENT SPICES - curries, chilly, etc.
- GARLIC
- WHITE AND BROWN ONION
- PRESERVED (PICKLED) FOODS
- FRIED FOODS
- ANIMAL FATS
- PRESERVATIVES
- ANYTHING ARTIFICIAL OR CHEMICALLY PROCESSED –
Colors, white sugars and excessive salts for example, which includes foods containing them: chocolates, candy, sweets, cakes, chips, etc. There are alternatives that are better for your body!
- ANYTHING 'BLEACHED' –
Flour, sugar – has been chemically processed and foods containing these basics (white bread for example) are not offering very much nutritional value at all
- 'JUNK FOODS' –

Store bought 'fast food' – you will know exactly what that means, typically these options present very little nutritional content and are heavily processed and high in fats and salts
- ALCOHOL (CHEMICALLY PROCESSED 'HARD LIQUORS')
- DRUGS (contrary to your teenage thoughts, sex and drugs *don't* mix)
- CARBONATED BEVERAGES (SOFT DRINKS)
- FRUIT 'JUICES' / 'DRINKS' –
Always check the label – anything UHT/tetra pack is processed, artificially sweetened and more often than not won't contain anywhere near 100% real juice. Fresh juices are more expensive and will be found in the refrigerated section of the supermarket – even then, there's a lot of serious *crap*. Always check the bottle and remember that there's no substitute for freshly squeezed OJ at home

RED LIST

Balance Essential Foods

Your red list contains a general guide to the parts of your diet that you need to avoid when you're detoxing and on an average day consume in a harmonious balance with your yellow list. There's dietary essentials contained on this list, which you're not going to live without, but having a better understanding of the foods that will impact your sexual scent for example will make you more conscious of where you need to jump in and lessen the impact they may have.

- COFFEE AND TEA (CAFFEINE)
- RED ONION - it's milder than the plain colored sort
- RED MEATS
- FISH – more oily fish typically contain higher levels of omega 3's
- DAIRY – avoid full fat, always opt for the low fat option
- EGGS
- HIGH QUALITY NATURALLY FERMENTED BEERS AND SAKE are the best options when it comes to drinking alcohol

BLUE LIST

Positive Sexual Fitness Foods

The blue list is great for general sexual fitness and should be used most often towards the food choices you make on a daily basis. These foods are packed with must-have levels of zinc, antioxidants, L'Arginine, potassium, B-vitamins and Omega-3's to name a few and some of the sexual fitness friendly natural hormones and stimulants, that will be sure to give you a positive lease on your sex life.

- WHITE MEATS - CHICKEN, TURKEY
- NUTS - ALMONDS, PEANUTS, PINE NUTS, CASHEWS, WALNUTS HAZELNUTS, BRAZIL NUTS, PECAN NUTS
- PUMPKIN SEEDS, SUNFLOWER SEEDS, CHIA, HEMP, FLAXSEED, MACA ROOT, OATS AND WHEATGERM
- DARK CHOCOLATE – the more bitter and higher in cocoa-content (aim for more than 80%) the less sugars and unnecessary processed ingredients it contains

- WATERMELON	- POMEGRANATE
- BANANAS	- APRICOTS
- AVOCADO	- FIGS
- OYSTERS	- HONEY
- CELERY	- CUCUMBER
- GINGER	- GINSENG
- LEMONGRASS	- RASPBERRIES
- STRAWBERRIES	- PEACHES
- BASIL	- FRESH OR FROZEN BERRIES

- LICORICE – tastes like aniseed/star anise - the exception to the potent spices blacklist - *kind of*. It is a useful addition to your blue list, but remember a little goes a long way for those not terribly offended by the stuff! (And so as to not offend 'B', just in case)
- SPICES – Ceylon cinnamon, nutmeg, cloves are blue & yellow listers

Try honey instead - a natural sweetener that will positively tune your sexual fitness and break the bitterness of that first coffee in the morning!

YELLOW LIST

Positive Sexual Scent Foods

The yellow list contains the foods that will influence your sexual scent in the most positive way and should be used closely alongside your red list to keep a *tasty balance*

- GRAPES
- APPLE
- PEACH
- NECTARINES
- MANGO
- PARSLEY
- PEPPERMINT
- PUMPKIN
- KIWI
- POMEGRANATE
- PLUM
- GOOSEBERRY
- CRANBERRY
- GUAVA
- CHERRIES
(SWEET, SOUR, BLACK)
- PINEAPPLE
- PEAR
- APRICOTS
- MELONS
- CITRUS FRUITS
- CELERY
- CEYLON CINNAMON
- SWEET POTATO
- BERRIES
- LYCHEE
- DRAGONFRUIT
- AÇAI
- LOGANBERRY
- COCONUT

GREEN LIST

Detox Diet

The green list should be followed closely during the 'shock' and 'cleanse' phases of your detox - your 'detox diet'. This list contains fruits and vegetables that are high in chlorophyll - which lends itself to naturally cleansing toxins out of your body. Whilst this green list is a staple of the first 72 hours of your detox, it's important to keep a high intake of those things on this list you like best going forward - much like the yellow and red lists supplement each other, the green list will be your best hope in maintaining your body's natural balance. You're inevitably going to consume various levels of toxins in the foods that you eat - and helping your body process these in the course of a typical day is going to keep in check the process that you're undergoing throughout your detox.

- CUCUMBER
- GREEN CAPSICUM/PEPPER
- KIWI
- LETTUCE
- GREEN APPLE
- GREEN GRAPES
- ZUCCHINI
- LIME
- CELERY
- GREEN PEARS
- HONEYDEW MELON
- PARSLEY
- MINT
- BASIL
- WHEATGRASS

WHITE LIST

Hydrating Fruits And Vegetables

The combination of natural sugars, salts and minerals and high water content (above 90% in most cases) in fruits and vegetables on this list will provide for effective hydration during your detox and work positively towards your sexual fitness going forward. The fruits and vegetables on this white list are going to provide your body with *purely positive* hydration and nutrition — and you can't hope for much better than that!

- WATERMELON
- CUCUMBER
- ZUCCHINI
- CANTALOUPE
- CAPSICUM / BELL PEPPERS
- PEAR
- LETTUCE
- PINEAPPLE
- CELERY
- GRAPEFRUIT
- APPLE
- TOMATOES
- STRAWBERRIES
- CARROTS
- STARFRUIT

THE 'DIRTY DOZEN' AND THE 'CLEAN 15'

When you're consuming a diet rich in fresh fruit and vegetables, it's important not to overlook one of the biggest downsides to buying fresh produce – chemicals and pesticides that produce is sprayed with. Unless you're buying all organic, you need to be aware of which fruits and vegetables are most at risk of actually causing you to put harmful toxins into your body, when in fact all you're trying to do is pack your body full of positive nutrients. The Environmental Working Group (EWG) has put together these two lists to educate consumers on what you need to pay attention to. In the case of the 'dirty dozen' list, it's important to carefully wash each fruit and vegetable that you're buying from a commercially producing source – although it's going to be impossible to remove all the harmful chemicals that have been incorporated into the fruit and vegetables while they were growing. The best alternative is to stick to organic suppliers as much as possible with this list.

This summary of the two lists contains the fruit and vegetables that are on your blue, yellow and green and white lists (as you're not interested in the black list anyway). The first list has been presented in descending order as far as the pesticide residue frequency is concerned.

Check out the Environmental Working Group (2013). Shopper's Guide to Pesticides in Produce for more reading. This information was sourced from the EWG. Available online at: http://www.ewg.org/foodnews/summary/

THE 'DIRTY DOZEN'

- APPLES
- STRAWBERRIES
- GRAPES
- CELERY
- PEACHES
- CAPSICUM/PEPPERS
- NECTARINES
- CUCUMBERS
- CHERRY TOMATOES

THE 'CLEAN 15'

- SWEET CORN
- PINEAPPLE
- AVOCADO
- PAPAYA
- MANGOES
- KIWI FRUIT
- GRAPEFRUIT
- CANTALOUPE
- SWEET POTATOES
- MUSHROOMS

WHAT TO EXPECT 'DOWN THERE'

During your seven days, you should expect some changes to what usually goes on with your *urination* and *purging*. (let's give *purging* the once over it needs and then leave well alone – in this case it's referring to your body removing its toxins in a *semi-solid* waste form) Particularly between the 24-72 hour period, your body will be heavily processing and getting rid of these toxins, so whilst there's no need to be alarmed - you should at least know roughly what to expect and to keep a bathroom close-by! Here's a quick guide.

DAY 1 - NORMAL - By the 24-hour mark you body will begin to undergo purging.

DAY 2 - Urine is quite clear and doesn't smell largely due to the water you have been drinking, and will occur more frequently than day one. Purging in the 24-48 hour period should take place several times.

DAY 3 - Significant purge in the AM. Urine will be yellow in color in the AM if you went about having a cheat treat on the evening of day two. After that, it should resume a pale color and take place very frequently due to the high levels of water consumption.

DAY 4 - Continued high levels of urination (remember you're drinking about double of what your typical intake of water would be, so don't get caught out. As for the rest, expect several *movements* today, which is your body finishing up with the initial 'shock' and 'cleanse' from the first three days.

DAYS 5 - 7 - You will be resuming more organized eating patterns, which means that you should expect business as usual in most cases. As you're not going to be concentrating on many black or red list foods, your body is going to be processing all natural and simple nutrition sources, which will actually do your intestinal health and processes a lot of good.

DAY ONE - "SHOCK PHASE"

First Day Blues

AS FAR as introductions go, I think that 'detox' has been the *in thing* for some time now, and as a result saturated society so heavily, that I don't need to spend a second either summarizing it for you at the front end nor convincing you why this is the one that will solve all of the world's problems in seven days (besides the fact that it more than likely will address some of yours, if you're willing to make the effort). I will keep it as simple as letting the title and let the words on the pages that follow speak for themselves. It may not be as structured of an A-Z guide as some of the others, but it's a straight forward insight into my journey towards being 'A' great tasting playmate - containing all you really need to know to make it through the seven days and hopefully get it right. Life didn't come equipped with an instruction manual and these seven days don't really need one. Everything you need to know is somewhere in amongst my glasses of water and random cravings for a well poached egg. And the best part - next weekend you can go to town, and really show off how much of a sweet kid the past week has turned you into. Then, I'm sure that as far as both you and your playmate will discover, all that delayed gratification will have been worth waiting for after all.

EXPECTED ENERGY-MENTAL ALERTNESS-HUNGER LEVELS FOR DAY ONE

Your daily guide will contain the expected: energy, mental alertness and hunger levels for each day of your detox, so you know what to expect as far as your typical daily activities are concerned – and when to take it easy during your seven days. Each day is broken up into: morning, afternoon and evening, which reflects the three periods of the day typically associated with or around main meal times. Again, if your days are a little back to front, switch it around so that it fits with your schedule. An indicative level of: high or low will provide you with your expected levels.

Energy –
Morning: **high**
Afternoon: **low**
Evening: **high then low**

Mental Alertness –
Morning: **high**
Afternoon: **high then low**
Evening: **high**

Hunger –
Morning: **high**
Afternoon: **low**
Evening: **high then low**

Day one of your detox is based on three main goals:
One – *SHOCK*
Two – *FLUSH*
Three – *HYDRATE*

I. SHOCK - Start the process of shocking your body into disposing of its toxins naturally. It's a very simple process that involves completely cutting all food intake for twenty-four hours. (Ok, so perhaps it's not as extreme of a concept of eating as far as a swimsuit model is concerned - eat nothing and your agent will love you for it type of thing. But rather it's getting your body to love you for giving it a break, and in turn paying dividends on how good your scent, *amongst other things* can be later, as a result). Most importantly, *it's only twenty-four hours* - we're not talking about driving your body into an utterly famished state (to then be allowed to eat a cube of cheese type diet) here, it's a simple wake up call - to actually give your body the chance start doing what it should be doing.

The other important activity involved with the *Shock* phase actually involves *shocking* your life out of complacency – and getting rid of all the black list foods out of your life. This necessary step starts the night before day one and calls for you to empty your fridge, freezer (I'm sure it's due for a good wiping down) pantry, draws, cookie jars, (yep, you heard that right) desk drawers, glove box, pockets – and anywhere you have hidden stashes of everything that you won't be eating over the course of the next seven days. Anything you are going to need going forward you're going to be buying fresh. Blue list foods that you have tucked away are fine to stay there, but the first 60-72 hours are going to call for little other than fresh fruit and vegetables – so an empty fridge is going to be less of a headache than not and making good habits going forward is going to involve shopping daily, for fresh produce. Much like your second goal for today, *flushing* – you are aiming to achieve the mental process of *flushing* all the *crap* out of your life. Have you ever taken to your credit card with a pair of scissors? (not saying that I have! Or haven't..)Well it's a bit like that when it boils down to it. Take to that black list with a big pair of scissors (and a garbage bag may also be useful) and make some new personal resolutions as part of day one.

Think of this as a head start on your NY resolutions, or as the second chance draw for everything you didn't get right the first time!

It's not just about doing the right things when it comes to a successful detox effort, it largely has to do with doing the detox the right way. That's why stimulating your body organically will allow it to best deal with the outcome you're trying to achieve - because after all, your body knows best about what's actually going on in there. *Put simply*, that means that there's no need for any teas or pills or 10-step processes requiring a user guide to tell you what to do and when. This detox, much like the basic idea behind what it all involves has a much more natural approach. Each day will be based on three daily goals, highlighting the ideas behind what you're wanting to achieve in that 24-hour stage of your seven days; together with a simple suggested meal structure for the day. It really is that simple - and in most cases you can logically wrap your detox goals and meals around the typical course of an average day. So we are really talking organic and positive ways to make changes to your lifestyle for the better – and doing so in ways that you can continue to draw inspiration and motivation from, long after your seven days are over. The other main difference (and likely the most important one) - is learning about how to let your body do the work needed to detox, and helping to then maintain it in good form going forward. You are after all trying to make your body work for you in a more positive way, right? So you should be doing everything you can to support your body in its natural process of cleansing. Think of it as taking one for the team! Having tried other detoxes in the past, despite a whole lot of starving and even more drowning in a weeks worth of chili-citrus water type drinks, there was very little to be said for what to do with your body afterwards - which if you think about it is actually the other half of your success story, after you've managed to get through a detox in the first place.

2. FLUSH - Your body by literally drowning it in enough water to seriously kick-start those *lymph nodes* into the cleansing process that you are going to let your body undertake. The water is going to be key on day one to stimulating your body into flushing toxins. On a daily basis your body has become conditioned to achieving hydration from various sources. On a typical day that may be anything from tea and coffee to juices and carbonated beverages and of course there's alcohol, which we will get to later on. Now not all of this fluid intake is going to have positive effects on your hydration, and moreover may dehydrate and actually cause toxins to build up in your body. So in the spirit of detoxing, your goal with flushing your body on day one is to allow it to take a break from the fluids that may contribute to 'negative hydration' and become *immersed* in the good hydration. This will in turn provoke some of the side effects (toxins) of the not so great stuff you've been drinking to exit stage left and not hang around and continue to do any more damage than they may have already done.

3. HYDRATE - keeping your fluid intake up on day one is essential to both the cleaning process and your own wellbeing. As you are only going to be drinking water for most of day one, this process of constantly drinking is going to allow you to satisfy your behaviorally conditioned need to ingest and the physical action and psychological satisfaction that comes with that. Constantly drinking a lot of water will do the trick there, and in the least provide your stomach with some volume and substance - so that you're not feeling like you're running on empty all day. You should be drinking at least 2-3L of water in a typical day anyway, and when you're regularly exercising, it's not uncommon to down 1-2L during a workout alone - so 5L of water shouldn't come as much of a shock to you. That's about how much I've averaged to drink on day one (I think it was way beyond 6, but 5 is heaps!). If you're breaking that up into the three meal periods you're going to have on day one, then you're effectively aiming to hydrate your body with 1L per meal with a few glasses of water in between each. Now 1L is about 3-4 glasses, depending on what you have at home, but in a practical sense, it's two small (500ML) bottles of water. And you will know yourself that when you're thirsty, downing one of those small bottles is a no brainer. So getting through two really won't be the end of the world.

Here's some *drink for thought* - we could happily go through a super-sized cup of soft drink at the cinemas over the course of an hour-something long movie. Now depending on where in the world you are that can be bigger or smaller but let's say there's a L there - no brainer huh? So don't go telling yourself that a L of water is a lot to be drinking in one hit, as if it wasn't water, you probably wouldn't be thinking twice about it!

DAY ONE MEAL PLAN

BREAKFAST (MEAL ONE)
I+ L OF WATER (plus another I+ L in-between meals)

LUNCH (MEAL TWO)
I+ L OF WATER (plus another I+ L in-between meals)

DINNER (MEAL THREE)
I+ L OF WATER
A generous serving of a single green list fruit

'Going green' on day two will give you a better understanding of what's involved in chlorophyll and green fruits and vegetables and immerse you in the process of 'green day'. But in a nutshell - the chlorophyll contained in greens is the main reason greens are in fact green. Chlorophyll has very positive cleansing properties - which is why this makes for a perfect first food intake at the end of day one, to help kick start the detox (and the need to eat something) process. Green grapes are an excellent strategy here and as a rough guide, about IKG of grapes should do the trick. If you're feeling particularly gnawish, then a bit more than a kilo won't do you any harm.

WHITE FRUITS

More commonly referred to as *water fruits* are particularly beneficial in the process of detoxing. These fruits, which are high in water content, provide positive hydration of digestion. The water content is sufficient for effective digestion and flushing of toxins. They also provide a basic amount of carbs, which is enough to sustain the body in your minimal energy requirements, whilst allowing the body to successfully enter into the required catabolic process, (day two) which will begin the breaking down of fatty tissues and toxins.

A QUICK WORD ON LYMPH NODES
AND 'DRY BRUSHING'

The story behind toxins and lymph nodes is as logical as it is good to pay some attention to. Think of it as is the daily task that will help boost the effectiveness of your detox.

Lymph nodes are the glands located under your skin, concentrated in various parts of your body that are responsible for filtering a lot of the toxins that run through your body. Their healthy function is vital in the proper functioning of your immune system and body health as a whole. So in the spirit of trying our best to get rid of toxins, grab a coarse, natural brush to dry brush your body with and get some serious *lymphatic stimulation* going on. You should be able to purchase them online or at a health store or decent pharmacy. The key is to brush toward your chest, which is the area that the lymph drains into your bloodstream, allowing the kidneys to then filter the toxins out of your body. (so above the waist is going to be downward and inward and below the chest, upward!) Particularly focus around your groin, underarms and neck areas and repeat twice daily, before your shower - morning and night.

One of the other huge causes of toxin retention in our bodies is the clogging of our body's pores. Sweating is one of our body's natural ways to promote the effective release of toxins (have you ever considered why body odor gives off a foul stench at the best of times?) Using moisturizers on a regular basis, whilst healthy for the general condition of our skin, actually contributes to our pores becoming clogged in the first place. So first tip is to go without for the week, and give your skin a fair shot at actually letting those pores breathe (with the help of your trusty little brush); and second tip going forward, is to avoid using non-organic moisturizers. Supermarket shelves are literally lined with *kitsch* products packed with various 'benefits' but what you need to remember is to keep natural – same goes for what you put *into* your body as for what you put *onto* your body. And as with the foods you choose to eat, there are alternatives – and cost effective ones at that – to the products you use on your body. In the same way that you're going to begin to understand ways to avoid chemically processed foods, artificial preservatives, etc. – you really need to be a more informed consumer in the department of lotions, shampoos, shaving creams, soaps - the whole nine yards that you stock your bathroom with. In a nutshell – anything that has unnecessary chemically produced preservatives and byproducts and parabens should be condemned straight to your black list. It's no joke – it is so easy to poison your body from the outside, in – and there's just no point, when the whole genesis of what the cosmetics market has evolved into these days is largely 'eco, *organic and natural'*. While on that note, there needs to be some serious level of consumer-awareness present (as with foods, there's a lot of *crap* out there too), you're becoming a smarter shopper by starting to pay attention to what's actually written on labels now aren't you? And never forgetting that the internet is our best friend, when it comes to wanting to know more about that little something we don't seem to have a clue about. Knowing what to look out for and what to avoid can sometimes be half the success in the whole decision making process. Use pure plant oils and butters to hydrate the skin – almond, avocado, coconut, cacao - are all positive alternatives that will offer your skin the most valuable, natural benefits.

And as for your trusty little scrubbing brush, it's one of the simple things that you will do to kick start your detox and going forward should definitely continue a few times a week, to keep your body in check!

DAY ONE Detox notes...

Well after midnight, and I'm already 3 glasses of water down and thinking of some midnight snacks à la homemade peanut butter and celery sticks. Gnawish! Little left to do but to sleep it off and look forward to my jug of water for breakfast.

Now personal preferences toward breakfast are largely varied. There's no real wrong way to go about it, as long as you're packing in a healthy balance of proteins and carbs. Making the first meal of the day the most important one will generally mean you're off to a good start. Be that fruit and Greek yoghurt, Bircher muesli, cottage cheese and salmon on a bagel, poached eggs or simply a protein packed smoothie - it's that time of the day when on a sensory level you're going to be most receptive to whatever sweet or savory line up best describes you.

So waking up with no breakfast on the list, besides a generous helping of water may prove to be slightly challenging. But as I have discovered over the course of day one - the power of the mind can be quite an unstoppable force when put to good use. The trick is to keep yourself busy for as much of day one as possible! The body has an innate ability to not only survive but also to burn through energy reserves when you're running on empty. That indeed may sound contrary to what your first thoughts were - however I found myself to have surprisingly user-friendly energy levels for most of the day. Add to that the particular sharpness of the mind, when you're busying yourself with concentrating on tasks which seem particularly achievable when you're not focusing on whatever your next meal is, and it becomes refreshingly less strenuous as the day progresses. And how about lending a small thought towards the uncomfortably sizable population of the world's impoverished, for whom this is a daily reality? All of a sudden walking a couple of days in their shoes seems all the more personally fulfilling - alongside the ability to set yourself a mental challenge and stick to it. It's not an overly bad feeling. After all we do set ourselves achievable goals on a daily basis that we channel our energy towards pursuing. Think of day one as being no different to these goals, which we play with setting ourselves on any other day!

I found myself helping with a move out of the family attic for most of the afternoon, followed by a mini-landscaping stint, before finally needing to satisfy the urge to iron a few shirts - and come on, I haven't ironed nor felt the slightest need to since secondary school mandated that whole 'fresh-ironed shirts with tie pulled tight' business - so a good couple of years to say the least :P

Drinking heaps of water is crucial to keeping hydrated - which you must aim to do at such time when you're not eating, and your body is subsequently chipping away at the stored energy, whilst beginning the process of flushing out toxins. Mentally - drinking water constantly will help to fill the conditioned behavior of constantly eating or snacking (which if you're anything like me, replacing 3-4 meals a day + fresh and dried fruits, nuts, peanut butters, etc. in between - will be extremely helpful!) It will also put something in your stomach, so as to avoid the perception of emptiness adding unnecessary fuel to the fire.

So your meal for the day (let's call it dinner, for the sake of establishing a timeframe for what you will come to appreciate as being the day's big event) is quite simple - one single fruit, (the best part – you're free to choose any fruit from your green list – or any green fruit you're into for that case) served generously and wash it down with your jug of water.

Me and my detox buddy let loose on about three kilos of grapes, (as he put it, 'nature's popcorn' - funnily enough, there's some truth to that by about 7 o'clock at night!) which went down a real treat, and I found myself snacking on them for the remainder of the evening. In summary - it managed to do the trick. By no means was it the kind of 'stuffed' that you might typically associate with a T-bone steak on a bed of mash (yep I said it, but we were all thinking it) but it was far from 'miserable starving destitution' either. Somewhere in the range of a happy medium perhaps? Which let's face it - if we manage to achieve every so often, under some level of extremity - we're doing all right!

Coffee COFFEE...! *If you're anything of an avid coffee drinker like me, freshly ground beans are a part of my daily ritual (largely in excess if the recommended 2 cups a day in case you were wondering – but pretty sure I'm not alone there). Between the near orgasmic smell of a fresh pot in the kitchen every morning, to afternoon 'pick-me-ups', and the occasional glass of warm milk with shot of decaf before bed - plus any excuse to 'go out for a coffee' anywhere in-between, the thought of going without was one of my major underlying concerns when I woke up on day one (that tall glass of water just didn't seem to have the same effect when getting out of bed). It becomes one of those staples, which positively charges endorphins and* surrounds the day with a generally 'can-do' driven energy.

So does that mean that (dramatically) cutting the free-flow of coffee for a day or two will be an 'end of the world' type scenario? I certainly would like to think so - but alas, I've made it through my first 24 hours as I'm writing this - and much to my dismay, I'm neither poking my eyes out nor dead tired just yet. On the off chance that I do actually get up from the really, REALLY comfy couch I'm sitting on though, I will probably be asleep in bed in five minutes flat.

So energy levels are at this point in need of a good re-charge (and a lot more FRUIT tomorrow!)

The final run-down on coffee? You're going to think about it, probably a lot more often than you would otherwise, and at times an honest proclamation to the tune of I WOULD KILL FOR SOME FUCKING COFFEE will actually make you feel better about the situation and more than likely move on, in an attempt to prevent from working yourself up anymore than the situation really calls for.

Now that 8 hours sounds really good right about now. I will fill you in on every grueling bit of day two, as soon as I get through stuffing my face with some kiwis in the morning!

**Spent about an hour on the phone, talking about food and things I want to cook with some inspiration for simple and light meals that can be made from 'non-congestive' ingredients within a few days of getting through the first 72 hours. Leaves something to be said for the mental clarity of your motivation levels to get some positive changes happening going forward. The mind is a powerful tool – and it's a good sign that a mere 24 hours can get it to start working to your advantage!

DAY TWO - "GOING GREEN"

Going green for a day probably won't save the world, but your body will thank you for it!

EXPECTED ENERGY-MENTAL ALERTNESS-HUNGER LEVELS FOR DAY TWO

Energy –
Morning: *low then high*
Afternoon: *high*
Evening: *high then low*

Mental Alertness –
Morning: *high*
Afternoon: *high then low*
Evening: *high then low*

Hunger –
Morning: *low then high*
Afternoon: *low then high*
Evening: *high*

Day two of your detox is based on three main goals:
One – *SHOCK*
Two – *GO GREEN*
Three – *REPLENISH*

I. SHOCK - Continue the process undergone in day one "Shock phase" so as to stimulate the body to dispose of its toxins naturally

2. GO GREEN - by eating only green fruits and vegetables for day two. Dark green fruit and veg are nutrient packed and owe their color to chlorophyll - which is particularly beneficial to the detox process.

3. REPLENISH - Slowly introduce the body back into food, by eating a lot of green fruits and vegetables. (In theory you're allowed to eat as much as you want, split over your three meals, but in reality - you're not exactly going to *pig out* on a super salad now are you?)

DAY TWO MEAL PLAN

BREAKFAST
1+ L OF WATER (plus another 1+ L in-between meals)
A generous serving of your favorite green fruit
Wheatgrass shot

LUNCH
1+ L OF WATER (plus another 1+ L in-between meals)
A green smoothie

DINNER
1+ L OF WATER
A green salad
Wheatgrass shot

GREEN SMOOTHIE

Using your 'green list' prepare a smoothie, using a blender to quickly blend your ingredients into a liquid meal. You can make use of both fruit and vegetables by this stage of day two, as you will have passed the 36 hour mark in your detox, during which you have undergone the initial steps to shock your body, and you're entering into a day-long cleansing phase. During day two you're going to be taking advantage of the basic process of catabolism which your body will have entered into, together with the power of 'green' to really hit the toxins in your body hard, and undergo a very crucial second day of cleansing after the prep work you've done in your first 36 hours to shock your body. By this stage you basically have your body right where you want it to be, and with some serious *green* support you will be on the right track to successfully and productively making it through day two, and past the 48 hour mark, which is always the most challenging at the front end.

SUGGESTED GREEN SMOOTHIE RECIPE

Grab your blender and fill it to the brim with a great combination of green fruits and vegetables. Combining flavors that may not appear complementary to the naked eye may yield surprisingly pleasant results - so don't be afraid to try something new!

Try mixing:
- Green capsicum, kiwi, grapes, lime, celery, green apple and mint
- The result will be a green nutrient packed smoothie that's quite thick, but will go down a treat on a relatively empty stomach and you should find that your smoothie will be on the sweeter side of the taste scale, with a unique, however pleasant spicy and tart intensity to it - apple and grapes are a natural juice base, the kiwi is sweet and will help offset the bitterness of the celery, which when combined with the acidity of the citrus and spicy notes of the green capsicum and mint will lift remarkably well and balance the taste of the final product to what I think you will find yourself to be a pretty decent liquid meal.

GREEN SALAD

Using your 'green list' prepare a salad as your first solid meal in 48 hours. By this point into your detox you will be slowly entering into the replenishment phase which day three is based on, whilst harnessing the power of 'green' to continue to *cleanse, cleanse, cleanse* for the rest of day two. Prepare a generous serving of anything and everything green that you're in the mood for, season with lemon and eat to your heart's content! The high water content of your salad together with the greens you're eating will do you more good than bad, should you decide to stuff yourself. Get creative with your salad, on account of it likely being short of a few of the ingredients you would usually throw into the mix. For me, kiwi and green capsicum (bell peppers) were a really' good combination, and probably not something that you would consider trying!

SUGGESTED GREEN SALAD RECIPE

This time round, you're going to be eating your greens instead of drinking them - so creating as varied of a mix as possible and packing your salad full of everything green you're into, will make for a texture-centric and flavor-intensive mix. Don't be afraid to go large and spread your salad into two sittings. Your body will thank you for it!

Chop and add to a large serving bowl:
- Green capsicum, kiwi, cucumber, lettuce, celery, green pear, green apple, mint
- Season with a generous amount of fresh lime juice, mix and serve.

THE WAY OF WHEATGRASS

Wheatgrass is a rich and concentrated source of chlorophyll and can be grown at home quite easily. It's also readily available for purchase, which will allow you to always have it on hand and make use of it daily in your juices and smoothies - much in the same way that you would have fresh parsley, basil, mint, etc. sitting in the corner of the kitchen bench. Fresh herbs in the kitchen are a real plus in the way of packing that extra bit of green nutrition to your daily diet - simply having them on hand is half the trick. Whether wheatgrass that you're adding to your juicer daily, or basil and mint added to a salad, tea or stir-fry - it's an easy way to make for some more effortless healthy, everyday!

If you're going for the *wheatgrass shot* approach, there's little wheatgrass juicers available online – both manual and electric/automatic, depending on how you want to go about it.

HOW TO USE WHEATGRASS

It's easily incorporated into your juicer - by adding the blades of grass in with your other fruits and vegetables. The same goes for throwing the grass into your blender. It can be juiced solo too - if you prefer the 'wheatgrass shot' sort of approach. It tastes pretty earthy and grassy, as you may have expected (but surprisingly not unpleasant) - so be sure to play around with it first so you can get a better understanding of what it's going to do to impact the flavor of your favorite blend.

SO WHY *GREEN* AND
WHAT'S *CHLOROPHYLL* ANYWAY?

Your green list contains the fruits and veg that are packed full of chlorophyll - which lends itself to their green color. Now the reason why this is actually of great benefit to you in your first 72 hours is due to the toxin cleansing properties that chlorophyll contains. Packing your body with a strict and concentrated amount of greens is going to really kick-start your 'cleansing' process and put your detox on the right track.

Chlorophyll is a powerful blood cleanser and blood builder. By replenishing and increasing red blood cell count, together with increasing the flow of oxygen to our cells an effective natural antibacterial process occurs. The benefits? Enhanced energy levels and wellbeing and a stronger immune system. Increased blood flow and higher levels of oxygen helps the body cleanse itself of toxins (like heavy metals), removing them from the body by binding with the toxin and additionally stimulating the purging process. So in the current detox phase that you're in, chlorophyll is going to be your best friend on day two - and the benefits on improvement of digestive, circulatory and immune health make for all the more reason to include higher levels of chlorophyll in your diet, going forward.

DAY TWO Detox notes...

Less hungry than on day one when I woke up this morning.

By the time I've been out all day, I'm genuinely starving and the cravings have hit. And I'm not necessarily talking 'of out of your way to kill the detox' kind of food, it's more a genuine want to eat the basics - poached eggs, steamed fish - the type of detox-friendly food that kicks in on about day four. Tomorrow's menu steps it up to some tuna, which is a thought I'm happy holding onto at this point.

Energy levels have dropped right down, and I think my current state could best be described as 'jelly' - in that I have little motivation to move around or do anything really. I'm not usually one for afternoon naps, but on this occasion I think it will be a must.

The structure of these first couple of days will result in lost energy levels likely anywhere during the latter part of day two. As your body is slowly churning through whatever stored energy it has left, you will find that you will hit a wall at some stage. That's why it's important to have these two 'slow days' to yourself, where you can satisfy any sporadic bouts of energy to your heart's content, or on the other hand do absolutely nothing if and when you feel like it's game over. The trick is to use the first part of the day, typically from the time you wake up +/- 6 hours to channel all your productivity into any physically or mentally enduring tasks that you have on hand. That way you can allow yourself ample time to rest later on when you're most going to need it.

Much like day one, energy is concentrated on your activities of focus - so as long as you keep going, chances are that you will keep at it. As soon as you slow down though, your body will have very successfully achieved its optimal catabolic state, resulting in the need to allow it to rest.

CATABOLISM is the process by which the body breaks down its own tissues for fuel, and this can be one of two things - fatty tissue or muscle tissue. General daily activities and light exercise will result in the fatty tissues being broken down successfully, during periods of minimal food intake. This is the *stored energy* that your body is effectively depending on to make do when you're not feeding your body at a normal, steady pace. (Take weight-loss 101 into consideration for a second - one of its main goals is this process of catabolism, in which fatty tissue is being broken down by the body, whilst undergoing light, however active exercise, while making sure that food consumption, 'energy intake' is kept low.) So in a similar way, as the fatty tissues are broken down during a weight-loss period, toxins are also broken down, and subsequently removed from the body - as they are no longer being stored.

You should however avoid high levels of physical exertion at all costs - largely due to the second process involved in catabolism - the breaking down of muscle tissue. During periods of *light exercise* (average daily physical activities such as walking, running around at home/work) it's the fatty tissue that's broken down to accommodate your body's need for energy. Heavy physical labor or concentrated exercise on the other hand will lead to the muscle tissues being broken down as the body catabolizes it's own tissues - and that can be pretty bad for you.

In summary - the body will always break down fatty tissues first during periods of lowered food intake, once these stores are exhausted, the body will begin to break down lean tissue and muscle as a source of fuel. Therefore keeping your energy output to a moderate level at best will ensure that you're not doing any damage to your body, whilst you're working to cleanse toxins and actually do your body a favor.

SUGGESTED PHYSICAL ACTIVITY DURING THE 24-96 HOUR PERIOD OF YOUR DETOX:

- Walking
- Jogging
- Typical daily activities at work/home (not including serious physical labor)
- A simple bike ride
- Yoga themed exercise (which becomes part of your detox today and is explained below)
- A swim (not talking laps here, just some casual time in the pool/at the beach)
- Mowing the lawn (if you have a garden and grass that needs cutting, it's a great time to do it)
- A light game of football/one-on-one basketball/beach volleyball — sports that can be played for short periods of time, at mid-range intensities. You should have a general idea of what you can do with your body without going overboard — so just stick to those activities and take it easy
- Light and easygoing watersports (jet skiing, stand up paddle boarding)

LIST OF ACTIVITIES TO AVOID:

- Heavy gym workouts (body building, muscle work, etc.)
- Running/sprinting
- High intensity sports
- Any physical labor activities at home/work (heavy lifting, etc.)
- Activities that may be dependent on high levels of mental alertness (remember you're going to go through peaks and troughs on days two, three and four)

YOGA AND LIGHT EXERCISE – A BASIC GUIDE

Much like dry scrubbing is going to help with your cleansing by stimulating your lymph nodes, light exercise – particularly during days two to four is going to boost your circulation levels further. The increased levels of blood flow, while you're taking proactive steps within the first 72 hours to *shock* and *cleanse* will increase the effectiveness of the process. As light exercise is the basis of the level of physical activity you're trying to maintain for the first few days of your detox, a 10-15 minute set of some basic yoga exercises is the ideal way to get those juices flowing. The AM is the best time to give this a shot, and if your energy levels are still reasonable by the end of the day, a second round in the PM is highly recommended too.

Start by grabbing some water and a small towel (not to suggest that you're going to be sweating profusely during your yoga routine, but it's good to have one on hand) and either a yoga mat (which is great for hard surfaces, beach and grass) or place a larger (beach) towel on a spot of soft carpet (the mat has to do with creating a comfortable surface to exercise on but just like the large towel, offers you a bit of hygiene). If you don't have a yoga mat, don't stress too much and stick with the carpet and the beach towel. Purchasing a yoga mat however won't break the bank (I found rubber mats on Amazon for around 30 bucks) and will come in handy again. Often, the purpose driven psychology behind purchasing one and having one at home, will raise your motivation levels to make use of your investment - even if it only is 10 minutes a day, a few times a week - that's all it takes really. Stay away from PVC mats – they are made from harmful chemicals, are unable to be recycled and leave a nasty little carbon footprint. If you want something completely green – your best choice would be a fair-trade organic cotton or hemp yoga mat. And finally – let's try this simple 10-minute routine of exercises. There's two basic sets of five exercises to start (each with extensions that focus on stretching muscles that get used during sex!) – **A** and **B** to cover the bases for both playmates, A being a top/active-centric set and B providing a basic introduction to the other playmate's core strengths. It's recommended you work through A first, before moving onto B.

Tips:

- Find a comfortable space to exercise in,
- Find the starting position for your set and work through the position and extensions slowly to stretch, relax and find your center of gravity,
- Work through each following exercise at a slow pace and concentrate on your form, rather than the speed at which you're working through them,
- Start with the basics, at least for the first couple of times and work your way through to the more difficult exercises. It's all about finding a good balance to allow you to get into a position and hold it there comfortably for 20-30 seconds. If at first you don't succeed – try again and hold for shorter times and condition your body to getting into some positions you may not have necessarily been in before!
- Progress through each set of exercises in the logical order they are designed to be practiced in - you will notice that your body naturally flows from one position to the next,
- Hold each position for 20-30 seconds,
- Remember to breathe – the trick to yoga is to let your stomach fill with air each time you draw a deep breath - that means you're pushing your stomach out, as you're sucking air in – which is actually the most effective way to breathe, as it uses the bottom half of your lungs and effectively utilizes your diaphragm. By doing so, you're allowing much greater amounts of oxygen into your body, which is key to every level of your sexual fitness. It can also be a simple tool for effective stress relief! Practice this breathing technique by inhaling through your nose, and exhaling through your mouth on your yoga mat for the first couple of minutes (in the Savasana position) before you get started, by which time you should have your new 'correct' breathing technique nailed!
- As a general guide to practicing new yoga exercises – inhale first, as you're moving into a new position or extension, taking a deep breath each time as you're moving into the next one – once you successfully hit the position you're after, then hold for 20-30 seconds and continue to breathe. Each inhale/exhale pair should last approximately 10 seconds. If you get around that mark you know you're getting a good amount of oxygen into your body.

- Each set of 5 exercises should take you 5-10 minutes. It's recommended that on your first day of yoga, you work through A Set twice, before moving into B Set. Once you have completed either A Set twice or both *A* and *B* Sets, you will have comfortably hit your 10 minutes. That *wasn't so bad, was it?*

- *AND* most importantly don't forget that *slow and steady wins the race!* Exercise to your own ability and don't push yourself further than you're comfortable doing the first time around. Exercise when nobody's watching if you're unsure – this is your body and your time, and privacy comes with greater comfort to get to know your own body better and gradually ease into trying new things! Keep in mind that these two basic sets have been designed not to stress you out too much. Good luck.

YOGA 'A' SET TO GET YOU STARTED

1. Savasana *(with 2 extensions)*
2. Goddess Pose *(with 1 extension)*
3. Supine Twist *(left and right)*
4. Bridge *(with 2 extensions)*
5. Boat

YOGA 'B' SET TO EXTEND YOU FURTHER

1. Child Pose *(with 1 extensions)*
2. Cat/Dog *(with 1 extensions)*
3. Cobra/Up Facing Dog *(with 1 extension)*
4. Plank *(with 2 extensions)*
5. Down Facing Dog *(with 1 extension)*

Yoga 'A' Set

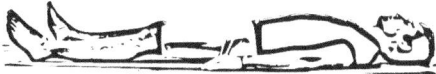
Savasana

Extensions:
1. Inhale, raise arms above/behind. Exhale for reverse
2. Inhale, butterfly arms up. Exhale for reverse/down.

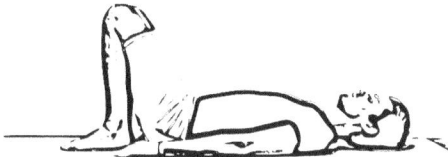
Goddess Pose

Extensions:
1. Inhale, keeping your feet together, spread legs/knees wide apart. Exhale for reverse.

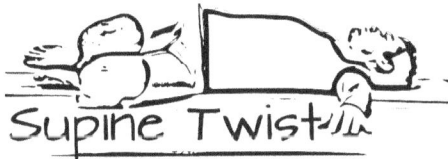
Supine Twist

Extensions:
1. Inhale, twist legs to the other side while keeping back/head flat + exhale. Hold for several breathing pairs.

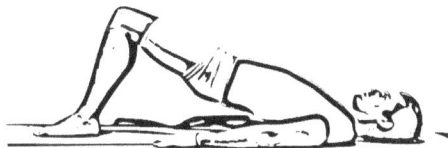
Bridge

Extensions:
1. Inhale, keeping your feet together, spread legs/knees wide apart. Exhale for reverse.
2. As above, except spread legs to shoulder width apart.

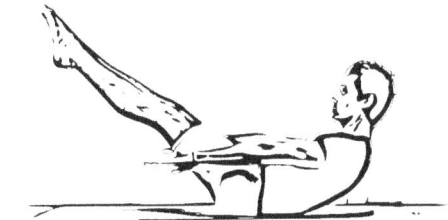
Boat

Note:
Inhale as you move into this position, hold for several breathing pairs and exhale back into Savasana to finish.

Yoga 'B' Set

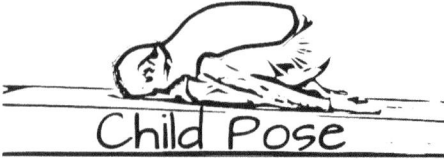
Child Pose

Extensions:
1. Inhale, butterfly/stretch arms around/infront. Exhale for reverse.

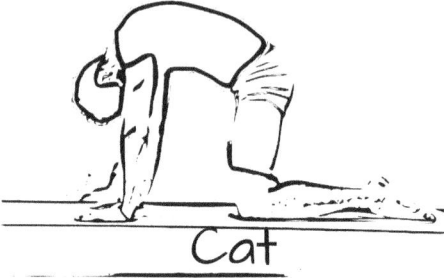
Cat

Extensions

1. Inhale, push your butt up and out (doggy style) and raise your head (your back will drop). Hold for several breathing pairs + inhale to return to original position.

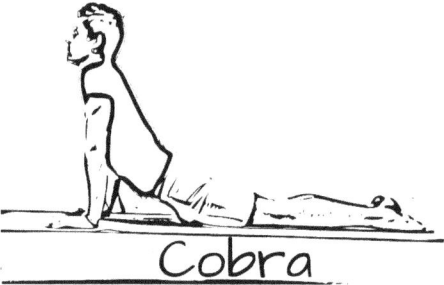
Cobra

Extensions:
1. Inhale, spread legs wide apart while keeping good form + exhale. Hold for several breathing pairs.

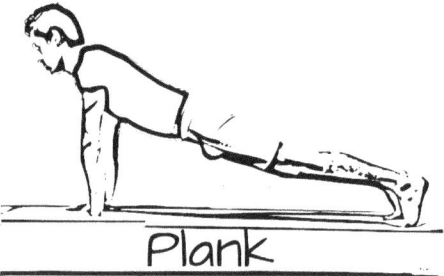
Plank

Extensions:
1. Inhale, raise one leg straight up. Exhale for reverse
2. Repeat several times, alternating legs.

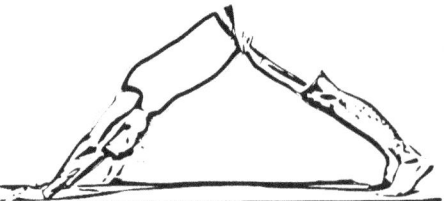
Down facinG doG

Extensions:
1. Inhale, spread legs wide apart while keeping good form + exhale. Hold for several breathing pairs and exhale back into Child Pose to finish.

So by the end of day two, you've successfully hit the 48-hour mark. This is the minimum period of time that's needed to allow your body to undergo its initial shock and 'purge' so to speak. What that ultimately means is that your metabolism will have reached it's optimal catabolic state, and has been breaking down your fatty cells and toxins alike, which has successfully started the process that you have been aiming for.

As with all goals in life, when hitting milestones along your way to achieving them you need to pat yourself on the back and treat yourself to encourage further progress. By the 48-hour mark, you will have realized that your senses are heightened and your body is craving all kinds of things that are usually part of your diet. In my case, black coffee was my *detox cheat-treat.*

Coffee..COFFEE...! *On the evening of day two me and my detox buddy flicked on the espresso machine and filed around impatiently, waiting for the thing to warm up and spit out a share cup. By this point, I can honestly say that I had such a clean palette that deciding on a couple of sips of fresh espresso was one of the most rewarding things I had done in a long time. The intensity and roundedness of this simple pleasure seriously hit the nail on the head. It's that whole thing about how you never know what you have until it's gone - so try to make the most out of appreciating the small things in life - like coffee, because when you haven't had it for 48 hours, honestly - it's enough to set the world on fire in my books!*

DONT FORGET TO DRINK PLENTY OF WATER around your detox cheat-treat on day two, to allow your body to continue to detox, and effectively flush this small intake of toxins by morning.

DON'T 'treat' yourself with anything on your red list (with the exception of a caffeine loaded drink such as tea or coffee). This is meant to be a small 'pick me up' and something as simple as caffeine is fine in a small dose. You do not want to disrupt the natural cleansing process that your body is undergoing and you definitely want to stay away from all non-organic solids when you're already a third of the way into your detox!

Caffeine as a detox cheat-treat in a small cup of tea of coffee is a relatively inoffensive toxin to break down overnight, as it does not contain levels of carbs or sugars which may be complex in nature and distract the body's heightened level of digestion as achieved in the past 48 hours. Caffeine generally acts as a stimulant (and is often used in weight loss related detox plans) so rather than potentially impairing the detox process it will both help your mental alertness and digestion process, while providing you with a much deserved pick me up! (while the water you drink afterwards, will help take care of the rest)

CUM (TO YOUR HEART'S CONTENT)

Yep you heard me right – think of these first few days of your detox as your *hall pass*. You are after all detoxing, right? And your cum contains toxins in it, just like any other bodily fluid. And thinking of this as a necessary part of your detox should make it all the more *purpose driven*. Seeing how this is a *Sex Detox*, I shouldn't be too concerned about too much political incorrectness when I say that *getting rid of a few loads* while your shocking, flushing and hydrate-overloading will basically be a good thing. So gear up, spend the evening in and prepare for spending the day *distracting yourself* tomorrow. In between those books and TV shows – you're bound to be able to find some that you will…okay I'm just going to go ahead and say it, *really get off to!*

DAY THREE - "CATCH UP"

Your day off to catch up on those books and TV shows you've been ignoring

EXPECTED ENERGY-MENTAL ALERTNESS-HUNGER LEVELS FOR DAY THREE

Energy –
Morning: **low then high**
Afternoon: **low**
Evening: **low**

Mental Alertness –
Morning: **high**
Afternoon: **high then low**
Evening: **low**

Hunger –
Morning: **high**
Afternoon: **high then low**
Evening: **high**

Day three of your detox is based on three main goals:
One – *STAY GREEN + HYDRATE*
Two – *SEXUAL FITNESS ESTABLISHMENT PHASE*
Three – *TAKE IT EASY*

I. STAY GREEN + HYDRATE - Continue the process undergone in day two "going green" to positively sustain the cleansing efforts achieved by your 'green day' while entering into the replenishment phase of your detox by gradually introducing the body to a solid and high nutrient protein source. Continue to hydrate, hydrate, hydrate!

2. SEXUAL FITNESS ESTABLISHMENT PHASE - Entering into the 'sexual health establishment' phase of your detox. You have had the opportunity in the past 60 hours to give the cleanse phase a really good go, so now it's prime time to start putting some rich and tasty nutrients back in there, as it will be the optimal period for your body to absorb every bit of good that you're going to be putting back into it. Day three will focus on the recovery of the physical aspect of your sexual fitness.

3. TAKE IT EASY - Slow down today and clear your schedule completely. The 60-72 hour period into your detox is the one during which your body will experience the most severe lapses in energy output you will have experienced so far. This is due to you having starved your body of required energy (food) intake in the past two and a half days in order to achieve your shock-cleanse phase, which, as you will experience first-hand will leave your body in a somewhat vegetative state. This is normal and to be expected, and should not cause you to freak out when you wake up in the morning, feeling like you've just had a huge night. In fact what you've experienced is two pretty big days in which your energy (output) levels have been much higher than the intake (rather than just one night of dancing your ass off for example, using the energy - sugars and carbs found in alcohol, to survive on). So two big days seem to trump one huge night in a really positive way, and you have every reason not to drag your ass out of bed.

Day three is definitely not a workday and probably the right day for you to just conveniently forget to charge your phone and just laze around in bed, catching up on all that TV you probably haven't been watching, while flicking through those books you know you haven't been reading!

DAY THREE MEAL PLAN

BREAKFAST
1+ L OF WATER (plus another 1+ L in-between meals)
A generous serving of your favorite green fruit or veg
Wheatgrass shot

LUNCH
1+ L OF WATER (plus another 1+ L in-between meals)
A tuna or chicken salad

SNACK
A LARGE GLASS OF WATERMELON + POMEGRANATE JUICE

DINNER
1+ L OF WATER
A generous serving of your favorite green fruit or veg
Wheatgrass shot

TUNA OR CHICKEN SALAD

Your first protein-based meal in 60 hours - and it will be the one that you have certainly been thinking about quite heavily for the past 24 at least. This will be a stage of psychological fulfillment, which you will understand as your body readily absorbs one of the core nutrition sources that it has been deprived of for the past three days. Halfway into day three, slowly introducing individual proteins back into your diet is also going to be a physical necessity, as your body will be running on a serious level of empty by this point and just as you have been hydrating extensively with water + your greens and white fruits, it's now time to start to put the right foods back into your body. The protein offered by tuna and chicken is very clean and simple and is most commonly used as a staple food (and protein source) in the diets of weight lifters body builders, athletes and anyone that spends a serious amount of time working on their fitness - due to the high level of clean nutrition that they offer recovering muscle tissue. A similar rhetoric does indeed apply here, as your body will by this point require some clean protein to provide a high dose of quality energy, to keep you going through to day four.

The timing of this meal is reasonably important - as a lunch meal you're going to be able to use it to provide your body with the required basic levels of energy to make it through the remainder of the day.

On a side note - eating a generous serving of a tuna salad today was quite phenomenal. Much like the appreciation for the 'cheat treat' cup of coffee I had on day two, the intensity of a protein on a virtually empty stomach was worth every bit of the wait. Not to suggest that I would be too interested in regularly going more than 60 hours without a decent feed, but talk about appreciating the simple things all over again. As you will see by the relative simplicity in the suggested recipe that I made use of, there's not really much to it, quite like your green salad on day two. And seriously, if this is how mind blowing a simple tuna salad is on day three, I'm so keen to get to day six, in which we begin to eat more complex protein and carb based meals.
PS. The BBQ the neighbors are having out the back somewhere is a little FRUSTRATING! (Keep your windows shut tight is all I can say)

SUGGESTED TUNA OR CHICKEN SALAD RECIPE

Chop and add to a large serving bowl:
- Red onion, green capsicum, lettuce, cucumber
- A 150-200g tin of tuna in spring water, drained (oil is out and brine contains high salt content). If you're going for the chicken option, grill (or poach) a skinned chicken breast on low heat (no oil) for about 10 minutes, or until tender
- Season with a lemon or lime and mix well

POMEGRANATE AND WATERMELON JUICE

Kick starting your sexual health is going to be a great success with the use of watermelon and pomegranate. These two ingredients are A-listers as far as their list of benefits toward giving your sex life a serious edge, and they offer some seriously cool benefits towards all aspects of your sexual fitness. Plus the two are a pretty decent tasting combination too.

POMEGRANATE promotes testosterone production in both guys and girls. Testosterone is responsible for sex drive in both sexes, together with being great for stress relief, which acts as a natural mood stimulant and promotes mental health. This superfood most importantly helps with blood circulation - which is key in the physical readiness toward an overall high level of sexual fitness. Pomegranate juice should ideally be pressed out of the fruit, using any old citrus press. If you have a large juice press on hand, this will give you virtually all the juice you're going to get out of this super fruit, but I found that using a standard electric citrus juicer (the same one I freshly squeeze a couple of KG of oranges with every morning) that does most of the work for you, is a perfectly suitable juicing method for this one. One note of caution though, it will spray a little so avoid staining the kitchen and yourself – pomegranate juice stains like a *SOAB.*

WATERMELON offers a similar spread of **++** reasons to drink up to your heart's content. The reason to love watermelons is the citrulline compound that the fruit is filled with. Your body converts citrulline to L'Arginine, which relaxes the blood vessels in your body basically enhancing circulation all round. What you want to aim for to get the most out of the citrulline watermelons have on offer is the rind (the green part) - particularly the light green and slightly soft area between the dark green skin and the pink flesh. You can easily scrape this with a spoon, which is preferable to actually juicing the whole watermelon, as you will find that the dark green skin is quite bitter due to the very high levels of chlorophyll contained. The bitterness in chlorophyll is contributed to by the presence of copper in its chemical make-up. However quickly peeling (slicing) most of the green 'skin' off the watermelon is fine too – if you're using a sharp knife, the process shouldn't take you too much longer than chopping and juicing the watermelon in the first place.

So the best thing about pomegranate and watermelon juice is that it's actually really simple to make. Juice a pomegranate and around a KG of watermelon + rind, and that should give you a few generous glass of this DIY at home *Viagra* mix to get you through the day.
Repeat daily.

SOAK AWAY ALL THAT BAD

So you're already familiar with sweat being one of the ways that your body rids itself of toxins, which makes tonight the perfect time to take a long, hot bath to wind down with, while giving your body an intense *sweat-fest* to successfully finish up day three's detoxing efforts.

As there's no moisturizing going on and the aim is to get those pores wide open and sweating, there's no need for any oils this bath time round. Instead try using a generous amount of natural mineral salts to make for both a relaxing and non-congestive soak. ½-1kg of natural mineral salts will do the trick, together with a few tablespoons of an organic spirulina powder – which has great cleansing properties.

Half an hour of sweating and soaking is more than enough – just don't fall asleep in the bathtub whatever you do – there's still a few days of your detox left for you to get through!

DAY THREE Detox notes...

If you're hanging out for a caffeine 'cheat-treat' towards the end of day three, you can go for it. Just remember to continue to drink heaps of water afterwards.

After a solid 10-hour sleep (and I mean solid - I don't think I even had the energy left to snore last night) the alarm clock rang, which was the first mistake for the day. This morning was a low point in terms of available energy I had to get up with. One of those typical mornings during which you snooze for well over an hour, before finally hauling (and I mean dragging!!) myself out of bed for some stupid work thing that should have taken place during the week. Within about 5 minutes of leaving the house, I was starting to find it seriously difficult to walk down the street, even downhill - so that required some level of motivation (and the off chance that the dog might actually be bothered enough to pull me behind her — she's only little, but always acts like a big dog, so if there was ever a time to put that attitude problem to good use, now was definitely it!). I didn't have the slightest issue with catching a cab home today (usually I would hate myself for being lazy enough not to walk the 5 minute cab ride). So I would strongly recommend actually not setting the alarm clock on day three and just letting your body do things at its own pace (if that means you sleep in until midday — do it!). You will hit a wall very quickly otherwise and self-exertion is not one of the three goals that you signed up for when you woke up on day three - let me stress that! Respecting your body is effectively why you've signed up for this 7-day challenge - and running on empty is neither sensible nor responsible towards the outcome of your detox and your own wellbeing! Bed and catch up on TV + books and that's it! (I mean come on - a guilt-free day off - you shouldn't need any more convincing than that)

By about 7 in the evening I am completely brain dead, and can't really move for that case. Staring at the evening sky turning all shades of pink seems about as meaningful as watching TV at this point - and as for reading anything, no comment. I seriously think that calling it a night by 8 (while it's still completely light outside being summer and all) sounds like just about the best idea I'm probably going to have left today. Might aim for a 12-hour sleep this time round!

DAY FOUR – 'BACK IN THE BLACK'

Getting back into the swing of things

EXPECTED ENERGY-MENTAL ALERTNESS-HUNGER LEVELS FOR DAY FOUR

Energy –
Morning: **high**
Afternoon: **high then low**
Evening: **high then low**

Mental Alertness –
Morning: **high**
Afternoon: **high**
Evening: **high**

Hunger –
Morning: **high then low**
Afternoon: **low**
Evening: **low**

Day four of your detox is based on three main goals:
One – *CLEANSE AND HYDRATE*
Two – *SEXUAL FITNESS ESTABLISHMENT PHASE*
Three – *FEED YOUR BODY*

I. CLEANSE AND HYDRATE - Continuing the cleansing process of the detox by hydrating your body with at least 5L of water throughout day four and embrace the high levels of water consumption as a positive lifestyle change and a permanent fixture in your daily routine going forward. By this stage of your detox you will be slowly expanding your daily menu to step outside of a strict 'green' diet, and as a result - you need to be really taking the hydration aspect of your seven days seriously. Whilst you're not going to be consuming a typical daily level of complex proteins, carbs, sugars, fats or salts during your detox, you're still flushing your body quite dramatically throughout, and most importantly - when you do transition back into a typical diet that will contain a balanced level of all food sources, drinking at least 2-3L of water daily will continue the process of maintaining your body in a good shape.

2. SEXUAL FITNESS ESTABLISHMENT PHASE - Take on board the 'sexual health establishment' phase quite seriously today, by jumping into your 'yellow list' headfirst. Today you will be focusing on not only the physical element of your sexual fitness, but your sexual scent too. The by the time you've reached the 84-96 hour period on day four your body's level of toxicity will have reduced significantly. As a general rule going forward in life, the first 48 hours are key in 'shocking' the toxins out of your body, with the objective of noticeably improving your sexual scent. So that's a good thing to keep in mind in preparation for date nights (and the probably more than necessary mid-summer palette cleansing you may want to do for playmate B's benefit). So it's as a result of the effort you've put into the previous three days, that day four is the perfect opportunity to start to sweeten the deal, by packing a whole lot of nature's sugars back into your body.

3. FEED YOUR BODY - Introduce your body back into a regular meal structure by preparing three simple and warm dishes. Begin snacking in between your two main meals, like you would during a typical day - whilst continuing to embrace a menu of a simple, single protein and a wider range of fresh fruit and vegetables. This is a key part of resuming your typical daily routine once more, and feeding your body with more regular levels of energy, in order to give you the ability to get back into the swing of things. By day five you should be ready to resume exercising and get through a full day without experiencing any impairing energy lapses, which would have been your biggest challenge throughout days two and three.

DAY FOUR MEAL PLAN

BREAKFAST
1+ L OF WATER (plus another 1+ L in-between meals)
Warm orange soup

LUNCH
1+ L OF WATER (plus another 1+ L in-between meals)
Steamed chicken and mushrooms

SNACK
A LARGE GLASS OF WATERMELON + POMEGRANATE JUICE
(With yellow list mixed in)

DINNER
1+ L OF WATER
Warm chicken and mushroom broth

SNACK
Fresh fruit jellies
Fresh fruit tea

WARM ORANGE SOUP RECIPE

This little recipe is as easy to make as it is enjoyable to eat – and will give day four a good, flavor packed start. You're over the halfway mark now, so it's time to start enjoying simple and wholesome foods again. Today's three main meals have been designed to create a flow of flavors, which will help you to replace things like salt, with some of the other flavors that you will have come to appreciate throughout the course of your day's meals, from one into the next. Leave about ¼ cup of apricots aside for lunch.

Add to a saucepan:
1. 1L of freshly squeezed orange juice
2. ½ a cup of cold water

3. ½ KG of apricots, cut in half and pitted

4. I teaspoon of grated ginger and nutmeg (plus try adding cinnamon or a clove)

5. 2 tablespoons of fresh lemon juice

Then boil on a low heat for about 15-20 minutes to allow it to do its soup thing and serve straight away, while it's still warm. Outside of your detox this is a great breakfast item, served slightly cooler with Greek yoghurt and some organic toasted muesli.

STEAMED CHICKEN AND MUSHROOM RECIPE

As you're not using salt during day four of your detox, this dish may seem a little less intense than usual – but using flavor rich fresh ingredients should make up for what's lacking in the salt department, at least enough to get by. Remember that your detox does involve cutting items such as salt out of your diet, so it's important to make the best of the basics that you have to work with. You're going to be using the water and chicken used to make this meal for the next one, so hold on to anything that's left.

You will need a large saucepan with a steamer tray inside:
1. Preheat a fan forced oven to 180C/350F

2. Add to the saucepan enough water to cover the bottom (about 2L)

3. Chop up a generous amount of lemongrass and ginger to add to the water, which will provide the flavor base for your steamed protein. Bring the steamer tray to a slow boil on a medium heat, which will allow all your flavors to start to do their thing.

4. Place 1KG of fresh mushrooms, thickly sliced onto the steamer tray, then place 1,5KG of skinless chicken breast pieces on top, and place in the oven for about 20 minutes

5. Prepare a simple sauce, using a cup of thinly chopped/sliced mushrooms, ¼ cup of apricots from your warm orange soup, ½ cup of your ginger and lemongrass water from the steamed chicken and some fresh thyme. Heat on low for 5 minutes and serve with your steamed chicken and mushrooms.

You can alternatively do the steaming on the stovetop too, cooking in the oven simply gives you a gentler steam, which I prefer to do

WARM CHICKEN AND MUSHROOM BROTH RECIPE

Using the lemongrass and ginger water you steamed your chicken with for lunch, together with some of the steamed chicken - you're going to make a simple broth for your third main meal.

Add to a saucepan:
1. The lemongrass and ginger water
2. ½ KG of chopped mushrooms
3. Pulled chicken from 2-3 of the steamed breasts
4. 2 julienned carrots, a cup of chopped celery and a handful of fresh parsley, chopped

Boil on low-medium heat for half an hour and serve hot, seasoning with fresh lemon juice.

FRESH FRUIT JELLIES RECIPE

This is a really simple one, and it offers as much nutritional value as it is not bad to eat – plus who doesn't like jellies?

You will need:
1. Agar – A natural plant-based gelatin alternative made from seaweed rather than animal bone marrow and skin. It has higher gelling properties and won't disrupt the cleansing process of your detox, with animal based byproducts, which you're avoiding during this seven days (and in general really).
2. 1-1,5 L of your day three juice blend (pomegranate and watermelon only) - so prepare this part of your juice first before adding the pineapple. to the remainder of what you're going to drink.

Pineapples (kiwis and papaya/paw-paw) contain an enzyme that prevents the gelatin from setting (bromelain) which means that your fruit jellies won't actually set. The way around this is to A - avoid the pineapple all together or B actually heat the pineapple juice on its own first to a temperature above 70C/158F, which should deactivate the enzymes that will spoil your jellies. This second option, whilst ambitious can get messy and it may take a few times to get it right - after messing around with it a bit myself, I came to the conclusion that pomegranate + watermelon will taste just as good and if you want to add in some orange juice or something like that, the jellies should set just fine.

What you will need to do:
1. Get an understanding of how agar works. As a rough guide 1 teaspoon of gelatin = 1 teaspoon agar powder. 1 cup of liquid will require 1 teaspoon of agar powder (or 2 teaspoons agar flakes *or* 1 agar bar). So depending on the amount of juice you're using, add the right amount of agar (1L would be around 3-4 teaspoons.

2. Heat your juice in a small pot/saucepan on low heat and dissolve the agar into the warm juice.

3. You will need to bring the liquid to a boil for a short time, in order for the setting to occur – note that unlike gelatin powder, agar does not thicken while hot, so don't stress if your liquid is still viscous (runny) at this stage.

4. When you've mixed all of your juice through all that's left is to place it into a baking paper lined baking tray (which will make it a world easier to get out afterward (and as we're not using spray oils this week, that's not an option, or molds for that case, which are just plain messy) and allow it to cool for about an hour, before placing into the fridge to set (which should take a couple of hours, depending on how cold you have your fridge set at).

5. Cover while cooling in the fridge. After the jellies have set, cut them up into small pieces and store in an airtight container in the fridge. They should be good for about a week.

DAY FOUR JUICE BLEND

So in addition to day three's watermelon and pomegranate juice mix, on day four you're going to sweeten the mix by adding some yellow list fruits, which are designed to be all about improving your sexual scent. Orange and pineapple are the suggested two yellow list fruits to add to the juicer today. Let's get to know them a little better:

ORANGE and citrus fruits in general are high quality yellow list fruits. The high levels off citric acid contained in anything citrus can help raise the PH associated with your sexual scent, which can contribute favorably to a better taste. Lower acidity levels will make for a more salted/bleached taste and the high level of natural sugars in citrus fruits will sweeten your success story, naturally.

PINEAPPLE That oldest story in the book about drinking a glass of pineapple juice to sweeten things up a bit actually does have its own merit. Pineapple in a similar fashion to citrus fruits lends itself to a positive sexual scent in that it is an acidic fruit. Acidic fruits have been shown to contribute favorably towards the bitter *alkalinity* present in your scent, this being the case with pineapple, much in the same way that an orange will sweeten you up. What's more, the naturally occurring sugars that are found in pineapples are PH neutral - which means that they won't throw your levels of acidity/alkalinity off balance, and in fact will more than likely do a few good things with sweetening things up down there.

All this scientific jargon aside — the jury is still out on all the 'hard facts' to do with all of the PH related stuff mentioned here. It could have something to do with the fact that the world of science is yet to commission a study that involves scientifically testing random samples of cum that participants are willing to drink and provide insight into as to the sweetness of sample A for example. Thankfully, this detox isn't about science — it's about what works! And the best truths often come from real people with real results!

DAY FOUR Detox notes...

Day four felt a little more on the normal side of the seven days so far. Energy levels were positive from the get go, due to the inclusion of a simple protein into yesterdays meal plan, which would account for the body having transitioned out of it's catabolic state and back into a regular nutritive cycle. As a result, I was able to have a great 10 hour sleep and start day four with a little more spring in my step - a great feeling considering how much of a slow day number three was. It's important to keep day four balanced as far as the level of physical activity you're getting yourself into. Your body is still going to be picking up from the first three days for most of day four, and it's important to not lose sight of the effort you've been putting into your body, by letting yourself basically go at your own pace for the day. That would mean more or less getting back into a typical working day and saving any higher levels of physical exertion for the following few. Light cardio based exercise like jumping on a bike for some fresh air is a good way to get out of your resting cycle for the past 48 hours.

Meal times were a highlight of the day. It was a more than pleasant experience enjoying some simply prepared chicken today, for both lunch and dinner. Having the ability to eat up a healthy and positively balanced set of meals gave my body the recharge it's needed for the past couple of days. That, combined with a wider variety of fruits (particularly bananas) made for a taste-rich day, whilst the higher overall level of food intake meant that the hunger situation was back under control. My stomach has noticeably shrunk in the past 84 -something hours, which meant was that I was actually eating less. This is a normal outcome to expect from reducing your food intake over a period of several days, and isn't any great cause for concern.

When considering this as being the optimal outcome for a weight loss cycle for example, it's actually a great way to establish a new pattern for your metabolism going forward. Eating less, more often is a healthier way to go!

On a side note, I received a frantic text message this afternoon from one of my GF's going something like this:
NIPPLES SO FKN SENSITVE!! NO BRA + MAJOR TEE RUBBING
LOL WHT2DO? ;P

Might that have something to do with the fact that she's a complete pomegranate and watermelon junkie since we both started drinking it a while back?

So let's broach the subject of coffee one more (last) time (as I know that I haven't yet mentioned it *yet* today)! If you're anything of an avid coffee drinker like is very strongly the case with both me and my detox buddy, this is one of the things that I have mentioned on several occasions as being perhaps a bit of a mood-killer. Stress not - it's time for a reality check on the subject. On an average day, drinking more than the likely necessary amount of coffee is indeed going to keep you perky as far as getting through the day is concerned, but don't forget that coffee is a toxin and it's one that's likened with producing some bitter aftertastes — not what you're trying to achieve here. But balancing it out with a lot of water and in a general sense not going out of your way to drink ten-something cups a day, means that you can mitigate the potential side effects coffee can have on your sexual scent. Like we are going to cover in the last three days of your detox, there's red list foods that you are not going to take out of your diet completely. So the more harmonious the balance you find between your red list and your blue, yellow and green lists after you get back into business as usual on day eight, the more positive the daily outcome of your sexual fitness is going to be as a whole.

The general purpose for having taken coffee off the menu temporarily during the first days of your detox has been to let the body shock, cleanse and purge - and coffee falling into the toxin category meant that it had to be put into the time out corner for a couple of days. By day four however and leading into the final three days of your detox, introducing a cup of coffee into your day is gradually going to allow your body to step back into it's typical routine. It's up to you whether you prefer your cup of coffee in the morning or as an afternoon pick me up. The morning option may have its perks for a number of reasons - together with acting as a stimulant at that time of the day when you're trying to get your juices flowing, the caffeine contained can work towards kick starting your metabolism for the day too (and as we know, a faster acting metabolism, as opposed to a slower one is a good thing! That's the reason coffee, due to its caffeine content has been used in a lot of diets designed to do just that). There are of course pros and cons to everything we do in life. The other side of drinking coffee on an empty stomach is that it kicks the production of hydrochloric acid in your stomach into overdrive, which can over time limit the body's natural ability to produce the stuff, actually counteracting the effects of speeding your metabolism by ultimately slowing digestion. Now end of the day, it's a personal thing and all we can do is take a look at both sides of the story sometimes and make a decision based on knowing all the facts. But as far as achieving the balance we need to in our daily lives, there's a lot of bad we can do to our body at the end of the day (which is the very reason we're sitting here and debating what we should/shouldn't be doing, half way through a detox). So the final word on coffee is that if you're into the stuff, then consuming it in moderation (in conjunction with plenty of water, of course) for the remainder of your detox is OK !

Dry Scrubbing – *Don't forget to continue to do this twice daily throughout your detox. Remember it helps to decongest your pores, process toxins and the general wellbeing of your circulation!*

And let's finish the day with some positive food for thought. You're at about the 100-hour mark now, which is well over half way through! (We're aiming for about 170 hours in total). The last three days are going to be heavily focused on the consolidation and maintenance of your sexual fitness, while putting together the building blocks for making new good habits going forward, as your transition out of your detox and back into your normal routine. There is going to be a few neat things you will pick up on, which should aim to give you some inspiration and a fresh set of eyes going forward, with ways that you can step up your daily routine and make a typical day's meals pack every little extra nutritional punch possible - whilst reinforcing that there's some things you just don't need in your diet going forward, and how to balance those essentials that you just can't live without. Day five, here we come!

DAY FIVE - 'ROCK HARD TASTE'

Staying on top of a rock solid lifestyle

is what your scent and fitness is all about

EXPECTED ENERGY-MENTAL ALERTNESS-HUNGER LEVELS FOR DAY FIVE

Energy –
Morning: *high*
Afternoon: *high then low*
Evening: *high*

Mental Alertness –
Morning: *low then high*
Afternoon: *high*
Evening: *high then low*

Hunger –
Morning: *high then low*
Afternoon: *high then low*
Evening: *high then low*

Day five of your detox is based on three main goals:
One – *LIFESTYLE ESTABLISHMENT PHASE*
Two – *SEXUAL FITNESS CONSOLIDATION PHASE*
Three – *HYDRATION + FITNESS CHALLENGE*

I. LIFESTYLE ESTABLISHMENT PHASE - Now that you have successfully 'shocked' and 'cleansed' over the past 110 hours your goal is to take your body back to where it needs to be. Day five is all about establishing your necessary nutrient balance and intake once more. You've started to introduce your body back into simple proteins and more regular meals + snacks again in day four, so let's keep that up by adding some more energy value to those meals and concentrating on those nutritious proteins and omegas (good fats) found in the healthy staples you can enjoy daily (such as eggs and avocados) slowly, to prepare your body for day six, when you're going to pack your diet full of these basics - which are great for both you and your sexual fitness.

2. SEXUAL FITNESS CONSOLIDATION PHASE – Having spent the past two days establishing your sexual fitness, day five is all about consolidating the work that you have done and training your body to adapt to these new eating habits that you have introduced it to. You have concentrated efforts on establishing both the physical aspect of your sexual fitness, together with your sexual scent and today you're going to continue doing both these things, by packing plenty of your blue and yellow lists into your meals and turning your new good habits into permanent fixtures going forward.

3. HYDRATION + FITNESS CHALLENGE - By jumping headfirst back into your typical daily routine, your levels of energy + mental alertness and general motivation should be right where you want them to be. Take today's challenge with a stride in your step by doing these two things, which should become embedded in your daily run sheet, in order to keep on top of your sexual fitness going forward.

HYDRATION - You're on the tail end of your seven days now, but keeping your fluid intake is as important as it was on day one. You've done the hard yards in your first three days - so it's a shame to let that go to waste now. Your body, as long as you are drinking serious amounts of L a day will keep up with the 'flushing' and 'cleansing' you have already allowed it to do - which is going to be crucial to the intake of more complex foods. You already know by now that this hydration will not only aid in digestion but also push as many toxins back out of your body as possible, after you've put them in. So if there's anything that you take with you out of these seven days it needs to be that!

Find yourself a IL bottle you're comfortable to carry around with you at all times, and treat it like your keys and phone - everywhere you go, the water goes. If there was a way to attach the bottle to your phone, I would be sure to tell you (surprised they haven't created an app for *that* yet) but I guess that's why we are calling this part of your seven days the hydration 'challenge'. Drinking water should become second nature, and you will fast realize that not drinking as much as you should be, will cause your body to settle back into the same complacent phase it was in prior to starting your seven days. All you need to do is keep an eye on the color of your urine – if it starts to darken in color and become noticeably more potent in scent – you will know you need to up the hydration.

So in summary here are the basic rules of your hydration challenge - keep your IL bottle with you at all times, make sure it's *refilled* at least four times and don't allow your bottle to sit around empty. If it's empty you're more than likely not going to carry it around with you and a full bottle will mean that you will more often than not sip on it, without even thinking about it.

FITNESS - The second part of today's challenge is physical activity, which as we know is another one of those several key pieces of the puzzle that we have been chipping away at over the last four days. You should have become comfortable with your basic yoga exercises by now and one part of this challenge is going to involve consolidating both 'A' and 'B' Sets by working through both in one sitting. The other part of this challenge is going to mean different things for each of us, which is fine - we all like doing exercise our own way (and some of us don't like it at all, which I get too) but as we have determined, it's never too late to start, which is why we have already given our detox a good go and successfully made it through to day five. If you're a naturally active person (be that cardio, gym, water sports, anything outdoors) then take an hour out of your day and do it. Whether that means getting your way around a slightly longer lunch break or a head start on your day in the morning, think of it as the *you time* both you and your body need by this stage in your seven days to really get your body back to it's former glory and most importantly, break a sweat so you can keep pushing those toxins out. Increased levels of physical activity during days five, six and seven are going to do really positive things for your metabolism. At a time when you're going to be pushing your metabolism more, your body is going to be as dependent on the physical as it is on the hydration. This serves to teach us the importance of balance in our dietary choices moving forward, as we become ordinarily predisposed to coming into contact with food and drink choices that will impact on our sexual fitness.

If however physical activity hasn't really been your thing, then taking few simple measures to change that can be surprisingly easy and will be all the more beneficial to you as you will quickly realize. Take your everyday physical activities on board and go the extra mile (and I mean that literally). Walking the dog or riding your bike? Now is a great time to explore a new route or track and get out for at least 30 minutes to an hour. Break it up by incorporating natural terrains into your time outside and you will be surprised how satisfying a beach, forest or lake can be. Challenge yourself by combining walking with jogging and/or running (the dog will be sure to love you for it), or if you're riding a bike - taking a track with a couple of hills on will be really refreshing after you've made it up to the top - while riding on the wet sand along the edge of the waves can be a great way to push yourself too. If you haven't tried it, it's definitely a must - dawn and dusk can be quite visually stunning times to be outdoors - so getting active early mornings or early evenings comes highly recommended - in the AM it's a positive way to get your juices flowing first up and in the PM, a genuinely *head-clearing* way to wind down from the day. If you're into SUP boarding or kayaking (which I both love) hit the ocean on a reasonably calm day and let the light waves give you a more challenging workout, which is great for overall endurance and core strength. Don't be afraid to check out your local gym or swimming pool either. For those self-conscious, (which come on, we all are when we haven't been before) there are times of the day when these recreational centers are less busy than others (peak times are usually mornings, evenings and Saturdays), so aim for your visits to be somewhere in between usual "work hours" when there won't be too many prying eyes there to put you off. Truth be told though, if you pick the right little gym for example, its members will usually be far more concentrated on their own workout than yours. It's a mental thing I know (and we all go through it) but if there's one useful piece of advice on offer - don't *psych* yourself out too much, people generally don't worry too much about what's going on around them. Rest assured though, that if something does get out of hand and goes wrong, in most cases there will always be someone around to help you out. Think of gyms as little *communities* - while there does exist a lot of *keeping to ones self*, there seems to be an unwritten rule between members, that they always have each other's backs. The biggest challenge can be actually making the first move (as with so many things in life). So even if it's nothing more than an innocent 'tour' so you can get a feel for the place, or making use of the free day pass for new members that most good gyms in the world will offer (even if that's spent on the exercise bike in the back corner, nervously watching everyone else) that's ok, you always need to start somewhere! What's the worst that can happen? You might actually realize that you don't mind it.

DAY FIVE MEAL PLAN

BREAKFAST
1+ L OF WATER (plus another 1+ L in-between meals)
2 poached eggs on avocado
A Small cup of coffee/tea

Remember – don't use sugar - use honey if you need it and a small amount of low fat milk is fine

LUNCH
1+ L OF WATER (plus another 1+ L in-between meals)
Whole-wheat crackers with cold roast meat + tomato

SNACK
A LARGE GLASS OF WATERMELON + POMEGRANATE JUICE
(With yellow list mixed in)
Fresh blue list fruit salad – combine bananas, berries, peach and anything else you feel like throwing into the mix.
A hard-boiled egg

DINNER
1+ L OF WATER
Steamed fish with tomatoes

SNACK
POPCORN
WARM FRUIT TEA

SUGGESTED DINNER RECIPE:
STEAMED WHITE FISH WITH CHERRY TOMATOES

Purchase a high quality fillet of white meat fish that has been boned and skinned.

Roughly 250-300 grams of fish should be enough per person.

1. You will be steaming the fish in the same way you did your chicken on day four. The fish should take about 15-20 minutes to steam.

2. Prepare a similar lemon, ginger and lemongrass water to steam with, and bring to the boil on a medium stovetop heat, before adding the fish and other ingredients to the steamer tray.

3. Arrange sliced lemon, dill and chopped parsley generously on top of the fish, to give it the most possible flavor without adding salt to the meal.

4. Surround the fish on the steamer tray with cherry tomatoes, which will be used as the vegetable side to the protein you're steaming.

5. Serve hot with a small amount of freshly ground pepper and fresh lemon juice.

POPCORN 101

Making popcorn at home is pretty straightforward – and it's a pretty neutral snack as far as carbs, fats and other nasties go. What's more, various health organizations around the world have considered it a '*healthy treat*', so it's no harm no foul as far as popcorn is concerned. Here are a few pointers:

1. Popcorn machines use *hot air* to do their thing, which is the healthiest approach – as you're not using any fats that way.

2. You can make it really easily using a saucepan and about a teaspoon of a natural plant oil – such as rice bran oil. Use about 50g at one time and make sure the saucepan is big enough to fill too halfway (about 3-4L), keep on low heat and leave the lid slightly ajar to allow the steam to escape. Once the popping drops below a few times a second, remove from the heat and empty into a large bowl to avoid burning the popcorn. The kernels are going to be pretty hot after it is ready so don't stuff your face too quickly.

3. Outside of your detox, using a small amount of salt to season the popcorn is fine - avoid using butter with your snack, as that's where this innocent snack suddenly becomes unhealthy and counterproductive. The alternative to butter is an organic natural spray oil – such as rice bran or olive, which will give the popcorn a similar coating to butter with a few sprays, which when tossed around with a small amount of salt will give you a tasty snack, less all the bad stuff. Also try other alternatives to salt like organic ginger powder, honey or paprika – depending on what you're in the mood for.

MAKING HYDRATION FUN AGAIN
SIMPLE FRUIT WATERS AND FRUIT TEAS

So you've flushed the hell out of your body over the past four days with enough water to probably half-fill a small bathtub. Let's keep on that positive note and take a look at ways to keep hydration interesting going forward. It's time to pull your blue and yellow lists apart and find ways that we can put those fruits and vegetables into some of the 5L of daily water intake. Your day is typically going to be made up of various forms of hydration - juices, hot drinks, smoothies and sports drinks, together with the water you're consuming everyday. So it's really important to not lose interest in water on its own, which may seem plain in comparison. There's a couple of simple things you can do to keep drinking water, while packing it full of the nutrients that you wouldn't necessarily consider eating otherwise. The skins of your favorite fruits are so rich and concentrated in nutrients, it almost seems a shame to just throw them after you've got to the good bits of the fruit you're actually going to eat. Fruit waters and teas are a great way to use the whole fruit. The process involves effectively slow boiling the fruit - skins and all, so as to extract all the nutrients that the fruit has to offer. The process of heating the fruit to a high temperature is obviously going to cause some carnage as far as *total nutritional content* is concerned, but on the flip side you're going to be releasing a whole lot of other nutrients from the fruit (that you wouldn't usually be getting any benefits out of) by using this very process - so it's not all bad. The key is to really take the slow-boiling part of the process seriously, so that you can try to achieve a happy balance, between getting some of the good stuff out of your skins, without actually nuking them completely. These waters and teas can basically make themselves on the stovetop, with minimal prep and stirring involved - so preparing a large batch in the evening for the next day or two isn't as complicated as it might seem! Once you have given these waters a try, get creative – put as many fruits and veg into the water as you can manage. Fruit and veg like carrots and avocado skins you probably wouldn't associate with a tea or water, but they won't cause any real grief as far as taste is concerned and the water will be filled with even more nutrients – which is a plus for anyone drinking it!

Purchasing fruit and vegetables that are slightly overripe is ok – they're only going to be boiled and thrown out when you strain. As a rough guide, you should know when your fruits and vegetables are finished boiling, when they sink to the bottom of the pot (roughly 1-1½ hours depending on the size of the pot, heat level, etc.) Once they hit the bottom, you can take the pot off the heat and let your tea/water cool. Remember the tea will taste different after it's cooled, so don't be too concerned with some flavors coming through when it's warm that resemble capsicum too much for example, as the intensity of these more prominent flavors will lessen once the tea/water cools. Adding fresh OJ (or one of your juice blends) to a chilled water or tea will also make for a refreshing drink.

CINNAMON 101

There are two main kinds of cinnamon: Ceylon & cassia. Ceylon cinnamon, otherwise known as cinnamon verum or *true cinnamon* is the only cinnamon you should have at home due to the low levels of *coumarin* it contains, and the fact that in its powdered form it actually tastes like real cinnamon. The coumarin contained in cassia (bark) cinnamon can be harmful to your liver and kidneys, which is an obvious reason for taking to all and any in the kitchen with that big black garbage back immediately.

As far as what's great about it – well both your blue and yellow lists would agree that not only will it help sweeten the deal, but offers a laundry list of positive sexual fitness benefits that relate to general health and hygiene. It's one of those superfoods that should be a regular and *must have* addition to your diet – and versatile to be added to anything you feel like having with it – sweet and savory alike. Try adding 1-2 quills of an organic Ceylon cinnamon to your teas/waters along with the rest of the fresh fruit/veg you're adding in there.
If you like to try new things – adding nutmeg and/or *(a small amount of)* star anise but surprisingly not unpleasant is not only going to pack some great blue and yellow list benefits into your teas/waters but also help you create some unique flavors that you may just end up liking.

BANANA AND KIWI WATER RECIPE

Banana peels are packed with potassium, lutein - an antioxidant that helps combat harmful UV rays from the sun (for those of us who just wont sit indoors on a sunny day), more fiber than the banana itself and tryptophan - an amino acid which can up your mood by increasing serotonin levels in your body. If that's not reason enough to hold onto those banana peels, then how about the simple fact that banana water can actually taste quite fresh - and break up the sometimes monotonous regiment of downing (or drowning!) yourself in 5 something L per day during your detox. Either way - it's worth giving it a shot! *Always remember to thoroughly wash all the fruit you're using!*

Add:
- 3-4L of cold water to a pot/saucepan that's big enough to hold at least 5L (avoid using hot tap water for cooking in general, to prevent trace elements of heavy metals getting caught up in your food!)
- 3-4 bananas, ends chopped off and cut into pieces (alternatively fruit cut up and peels thrown in whole, with ends cut off - always cut the ends off a banana peels and fruit in general, as that's where insects most commonly work away at the fruit) and always remove the stickers from the fruits (they may look cute, but sadly don't offer any nutritional value)
- 5 kiwis, chopped into pieces
- A small handful of fresh mint leaves
- Half a lemon, chopped (peel and all)
- I large cucumber, chopped (with ends cut off)
- A handful of grapes

Bring to the boil, then boil:
- For about an hour on a low heat, half covered, and then let sit for another hour with no heat.

Strain:
- After the water has cooled, strain into a jug (or a few jugs). You should have roughly 3 L of fruit water left. This is the part where you

get a feel for how your water tastes and what you can do to spice it up for tomorrow's effort. You're probably not going to be blown away by the taste intensity of the water (there's no sugar after all and it is a water, not a juice - but it's packed with a lot of nutrients that water alone isn't typically going to offer) but adding more fruit will fix that, and you will end up with more of a compote. You can always add honey, if you're into the whole sweet thing. You can place your water into the fridge, as it will taste perfectly acceptable chilled the next day.

GINGER, LEMONGRASS AND BERRY TEA RECIPE

Ginger, lemongrass and berries all rate well and are found on your blue list, so as far as teas go, this isn't a bad one to take a shot at. You can try adding some organic tea to the mix too — fruit/green/herb/jasmine etc. tea bags or loose leaf tea will make for a more rounded final flavor — try adding a few heaped tablespoons or 2-3 teabags to the pot.

Add:
- 3-4L of cold water to a pot/saucepan that's big enough to hold at least 5L
- A couple (2-4) thick slices of ginger (ginger is great for you and lends itself to being in a tea - it's a taste that may be unfriendly to some however so less can be more, whilst more is perfectly acceptable too)
- 1-2 stalks of lemongrass, chopped/smashed (same as with ginger - it's strong, so figure out how much is going to work for you)
- A cup of berries - strawberries, blueberries, blackberries, raspberries, cranberries - whatever you can get your hands on and enjoy the taste of. Each different berry is going to have a distinct tartness or sweetness to it - so find the one you like best.
- A small handful of fresh mint leaves
- A chopped lemon, the whole fruit + peel
- 2 chopped oranges, the whole fruit + peel
- A handful of apricots and a peach (seed and all)

Bring to the boil, then boil:
- For about an hour on a low heat, half covered, and then let sit for another hour with no heat.

Strain:
- After the tea has cooled, strain into a jug and sweeten with some honey. Adding honey to 'boiling' hot liquids will nuke a lot of its nutrients, whereas lukewarm liquids will just help dissolve the honey, and keep all the good intact. Your tea can be enjoyed both warm and cold (iced is great too). If you have fresh ginseng on hand (ginseng root, fresh or dried is accessible in a lot of fresh markets/supermarket chains now and you will almost always find it in Asian supermarkets too) adding some to your tea will pack some more blue list plus points into your tea!

RED AND YELLOW LIST FOODS

Your red list is made up of staples that are going to be a part of your daily life but as you know won't necessarily do your sexual scent any favors. Part of the consolidation of your sexual fitness is going to be developing a closer awareness of the need to balance these foods with your yellow list – which you have been working with closely on day five. As with all your newly formed habits going forward it's just a matter of getting to know your lists and even having them stuck to the fridge for a while as cheat sheets. It's a simple pattern to follow and it will become second nature after a while – so don't be too concerned if you're referring back to your lists constantly going forward, as that's what they are there for! All you need to do is take a broad view of the practical application of these lists to your daily meals – you already know all about hydration where coffee is concerned, to get those toxins back out again – the same goes for your sexual scent. Having a steak sandwich with lunch? Down a large glass of your *superfruitjuice* with it. Eating a lot of dairy? Have a pineapple, citrus and chopped mint fruit salad for dessert. It's all in the balance, and making more conscious choices and just plain *paying attention* are going to be your biggest assets going forward.

DAY SIX 'IN A NUTSHELL'

You will find not only a peanut, but also more of the good stuff than you can even imagine

EXPECTED ENERGY-MENTAL ALERTNESS-HUNGER LEVELS FOR DAY SIX

Energy –
Morning: **high**
Afternoon: **high then low**
Evening: **high**

Mental Alertness –
Morning: **low then high**
Afternoon: **high**
Evening: **high then low**

Hunger –
Morning: **high then low**
Afternoon: **high then low**
Evening: **high then low**

Day six of your detox is based on three main goals:
One – *LIFESTYLE CONSOLIDATION PHASE*
Two – *SEXUAL FITNESS MAINTENANCE PHASE*
Three – *NUTRITIONAL ORIENTATION*

I. LIFESTYLE CONSOLIDATION PHASE - Continue the 'lifestyle establishment' phase started on day five by packing your body full of the right kind of foods and use day six and seven to get a full grasp of these lifestyle choices you're consciously beginning to make. A solid appreciation of the *why* is half the success to the *doing it* going forward. Understand your black list at a time when you're getting ready to launch back into your normal routine, by finding the best alternatives to replace the foods that you're taking out of a typical day.

2. SEXUAL FITNESS MAINTENANCE PHASE – Days six and seven are going to get you working away at your blue list – which is going to be your best friend going forward with your new and improved sexual fitness.

3. NUTRITIONAL ORIENTATION - Get to know what you're actually feeding your body on a typical day. There's far too many choices when you hit the shelves of your local supermarket, and with that comes a lot of confusion and potentially bad choices. Understand more about where your black list foods may be hiding and how to make the most out of your red and blue list foods, without throwing your body's state of grace out of whack.

DAY SIX MEAL PLAN

BREAKFAST
1+ L OF WATER (plus another 1+ L in-between meals)
Cooked ham and eggs on a slice of whole-wheat bread
Freshly squeezed orange juice
A cup of coffee/tea

SNACK
LARGE GLASS WATERMELON + POMEGRANATE SMOOTHIE
(With yellow list mixed in)
Freshly made peanut butter and popcorn

LUNCH
1 + L OF WATER (plus another 1+ L in-between meals)
Whole-wheat crackers with either a natural (100% pork meat) ham, cold roast meat (corned beef for example is so good) or tuna, with lettuce, tomato, red onion, cucumber, grated carrot (you're in charge)

and lightly seasoned with salt and pepper (and lemon if you're in the mood)

SNACK
A LARGE GLASS OF WATERMELON + POMEGRANATE JUICE
(With yellow list mixed in)
Fresh fruit
A cup of coffee/tea
Celery and peanut butter sticks

DINNER
1+ L OF WATER
Asian style lemongrass chicken broth

SNACK
Popcorn
Choc-peanut butter ice-cream/whip
Fruit tea

L'ARGININE, OMEGA-3'S AND PEANUT BUTTER

Peanut butter, when made purely out of peanuts without any added salts, sugars of fats, rates highly on your blue list. When you're making it at home, it's a breeze to throw together any nut butter out of your favorite nut, or mix of nuts. Almonds, cashews, walnuts, hazelnuts, pine nuts, brazil nuts and pecans – to name a few are all going to help your sexual fitness go that extra mile. Nuts are a very rich source of L'Arginine, which is an essential amino acid that converts to Nitric Oxide in your body. This process results in the relaxation of blood vessels, causing greater blood flow through your body. Consuming high levels of L'Arginine has also been found to help stimulate additional growth hormone secretion, which is going to fare well for both your sexual fitness and a positively active lifestyle as a whole.
Omega-3's are next in line to add another thumbs up to peanut butter. Omega-3's are an essential fatty acid (which makes them the

good sort) that much like L'Arginine naturally occurs in your body. Research has suggested that this type of fatty acid is linked closely with increasing blood flow to those places that will count the most when you're getting to know your playmate, inside and out. Consuming foods that contain high levels of these essential acids - found on your blue list needs to become a part of the daily ritual of what you're putting into your body. Finding ways to add them to your diet can really be as painless as whipping up a simple peanut butter, and working your way through a couple of tablespoons a day. There's countless ways you can incorporate peanut butter into everyday snacking, recipes and eating and any number of various nut butters that can be made. And for those of you with peanut allergies, don't stress too much – there's plenty of other L'Arginine and Omega-3 packed foods on your blue list – try oats, flax and eggs. The great thing about the blue list is that it contains a wide variety of foods, which will be suited to all kinds of tastes, meals and nutritional requirements. Eggs are a red list food, but they lend themselves to being a blue list food also, as they are packed with Omega-3's as well as being a great protein source, so don't hold back on a few eggs in your daily diet, while keeping them well balanced.

HOW TO MAKE PEANUT BUTTER AT HOME

½ KG of peanuts (or any kind of nut) will make for a large jar, enough to last you a good part of a week (if you like the stuff as much as I do, don't be shy and make some more). If you're playing around with different nut butters, ¼ KG is enough to figure out whether your combination is a winner.

Always use a high quality, organic toasted nut (unsalted and definitely not fried) – remember that putting lower quality substitutes into anything you're eating, just means that you will be putting *crap* back into your body – and you haven't got this far to take two steps back, have you.

Add the peanuts to a food processor. Depending on the food processor you're using it may take more or less time - but as a rough guide, a 1500W engine should take 5 minutes to get you to where you want to be. Your peanut butter will pass through three stages from start to finish:

Stage 1: Nuts will become crushed and turn into a fine, flour-like powder.

Stage 2: The nuts will begin to release their natural oils and the powder mix will clump and turn into a sticky ball. At this point if you need to scrape the edges of your food processor, it's the right time to do it.

Stage 3: Upon further processing, the remainder of the oils binding the ball of butter will be released, at which point the peanut butter will become somewhat oily and more recognizable in consistency. By this stage you will continue to process for another 1-2 minutes to produce a smooth peanut butter.

If you like crunchy (like me) all you need to do is grind a handful of peanuts in a coffee grinder and throw them into the mixer for a couple of seconds, to combine with the smooth butter you've made.

Note that some of the nuts you may want to use will contain less naturally occurring oils than others, and you may need to add a small amount of one of your healthy oils to allow the nuts to actually get to the butter stage (without turning into a thick, dry paste). Alternatively mixing some of these nuts, with ones containing higher levels of naturally occurring oils is a good way to achieve the nut butter you're after, and save the oils for cooking instead

SUGGESTED PEANUT BUTTER CUPS RECIPE:

1. Melt a few blocks of a dark cocoa (85% +) chocolate on low heat
2. Prepare a fresh batch of peanut butter (with pinch of salt)
3. Pour 1-2 tablespoons chocolate into silicon muffin trays, together with 1-tablespoon peanut butter. Drizzle some extra chocolate on top *Allow to set in the fridge and indulge. These are so damn good.*

SUGGESTED DINNER RECIPE:
ASIAN STYLE LEMONGRASS CHICKEN BROTH

You will have become familiar with this type of soup on day four – so it shouldn't cause you too much grief to throw together. You've consumed a broader variety of foods today, and this light broth will be a light and well balanced third main meal for day six, and one that you can easily embellish in the future, for a simple, quick and healthy meal.

1. Add the usual suspects to a pot of water: lemongrass, ginger, chicken breasts, carrot and lemon. This time you will be stepping up the flavor a notch by incorporating a half-cup of a natural coconut milk and coriander/cilantro into the mix.

2. Simmer on a medium heat for about 20 minutes and serve in a large soup bowl with a handful of beansprouts thrown in. Season with fresh lemon juice and pepper.

CHOC-PEANUT BUTTER ICE-CREAM/WHIP RECIPE

Using your food processor once again, you're going to prepare a protein-friendly dessert, packed with some of the good stuff found in the peanut butter you have made. Slowly you're putting red listers back into your diet, and in this case you're going to go with a low fat cottage cheese or Greek yoghurt, providing you with some of the calcium and other nutrients found in dairy that your body needs introduced to your diet once again. If you're unsure which to use, as a general guide, cottage cheese will produce a more *fluffy* whip than Greek yoghurt, but may leave small traces of the curd, unless you're using a reasonably high powered mixer. As far as balance goes – you know the drill, and as you have packed your meals today full of your superfruits and yellow listers, the dairy hit isn't going to set you back as long as you're drinking a decent amount of your fruit tea or water to wash it down with, before bed.

1. Add 1 cup of low fat cottage cheese or low fat Greek yoghurt to your food processor, together with 2 tablespoons of your peanut butter, a frozen banana, 1 teaspoon of an organic cocoa powder and 1-2 tablespoons of honey to sweeten, depending on how sweet you're into.

2. Process on high until you achieve a mouse/whipped consistency. Now it's the first time you have had a chocolate-something in nearly a week, so enjoy it straight from the bowl, and freeze up whatever's left for a couple of hours until it reaches a frozen yogurt like state. Note that if you leave it frozen overnight, your mousse will likely become quite solid, leaving it in the fridge the next day for a couple of hours should get it back to where you want it to be.

You may need to make some more in order to get the mixer properly working, so simply refrigerating/freezing the rest and spreading it out as a snack for a couple of days is okay too.

CUTTING THE CRAP OUT OF YOUR DIET..

Means being a more conscientious, assertive and informed shopper. Knowing what to avoid is only half the success, as there is a lot of seriously low quality food available to the general public. Due to ultra relaxed food labeling regulations, (in virtually all parts of the world) a lot of sub-standard fresh and packaged produce makes its way onto the shelves, alongside its seemingly overpriced (but in reality, actually good for you) organic counterparts. The bottom line is that some of these 'low-cost' (and more often than not, eye-catching) products just aren't great for you and you should avoid the temptation to play the 'cheaper is better' game at all costs, when it comes to your nutrition and what you're putting into your body as a general rule.

So as part of day six's 'nutritional orientation', let's take a look at some of the most common foods you will eat daily so we can make an informed decision on what's actually good vs. what's not so great and buy the right things, which are going to be best for us.

EGGS – As you know eggs are a high source of a lot of the good things you want to be packing into your body everyday – so it's important to make sure that the eggs you're eating are the most healthy for you. Free-range, organic, grain fed eggs are the only real option worth considering. They will offer a natural and high nutritional value and none of the nasty stuff comes with a low priced egg. The moral of the story with foods that you eat is that you get what you pay for. Now that doesn't mean that you have to break the bank – which I would strongly advise against – don't get caught up in the three times the price foods labeled "bio" or organic, just because the label says so. Part of being an informed consumer is as you know, reading the labels and knowing what to look out for. There are a lot of body-friendly options available now all over the place, which will likely be marginally higher in price, but will actually resemble a more accurate market value pricing point, for what you should be paying for the product. As opposed to the extremely underinflated prices associated with low-cost products, that in turn present a perceivable, however unrealistic difference in price. It's a little bit to wrap your head around, but it makes good sense when you start looking around next time you shop. Back to your egg – be sure to look for options offering higher levels of Omega-3's (much like certain brands of fresh milk, offering higher levels of calcium for example). That's usually a good sign of a high quality product. Reality is with eggs, like most fresh produce – the better the animals producing the product are treated, the more friendly the product is going to be. So when you think about a cage-enclosed chicken, that's artificially fed and unlikely to be regulated by 'cruelty-free' living conditions - producing eggs reeking of stress and just bad everything, would you really want to be eating that kind of an egg? I'll pass on that, thanks.

HAMS (AND LUNCH MEATS) - So some of the main things you have tried to avoid throughout your detox include the very stuff that can be found inside your typical 'run of the mill' hams, conveniently found in each supermarket. For your information - most hams are actually processed, which means that you're eating something with *maybe* 80 percent of actual meat, the rest is made up on parts of the animal you don't even want to hear about. And that 80 percent number is a best case scenario, without even the mention of the tinned, preserved options also conveniently at your disposal. The rule of thumb with hams will not be dissimilar to everything else you will buy – a higher price, will generally reflect a higher and cleaner protein content, with less 'fillers' that generally contribute to a cheaper price. Avoid pastramis, chicken loaves and anything that's roughly half the price of what an average ham would be – as it's *shit* not even worth feeding to the dog, seriously. Forget about anything overly smoked, salamis are obviously out and anything that has been formed (round shaped hams, square shaped hams and you will know exactly what I mean when I say *smiley hams* – which feel about as greasy to touch on a good day, as ordinary ham that's about 3 days too old) has been processed, and molded using a process called 'tumbling', which is basically designed to make the ham look a lot better than what it actually is, so that's out of the question too. A natural ham, or roasted meat will resemble the shape of something that would actually come from the leg or shoulder of an animal, which makes perfect sense. So keep a serious eye out for bad hams (and 'lunch meats') as it's seriously not worth it.

CHICKEN, STEAKS, PORK AND CUTS OF MEAT – Much like the chicken and the egg, you need to get into the free-range, grain fed type situations, which involve the highest quality of meat produced as a result of the natural lifestyle that's offered prior to the chop-house. Look for cuts of meat that are trim (skin and fat free), fresh (definitely avoid buying frozen – if you want, you can do the freezing yourself, and know how long it's actually been like that for) and only ever buy from reputable butchers and supermarket chains that you can trust. Your general health is one thing, but food poisoning – that's a separate ball game you will just kick yourself for. It may all sound like pretty common sense stuff, which it is! So you should know all the better that paying attention to the small details will pay dividends in the long run.

BREADS – Are plenty, and equally not good if you're not buying the right stuff. Avoiding anything made from bleached flour is a given scratch off the list, and buying soft and fluffy sliced and colorfully packaged breads will usually bear a high content of artificial no-goods, which you want to avoid too. Dark whole wheat and rye breads are slightly dense in nature, due to being packed full of seeds - which are right at the top of your blue list, so a big *yes* there. Being concentrated with other ingredients besides flours and yeasts will mean the bread will contain a significantly lower level of carbs and a low *glycemic index* – meaning you won't be hungry five minutes after you've eaten, which *is* a good thing. The same whole wheat concept goes for crackers, crisp breads, flat breads, etc. For these types of breads, also avoid buying anything that has been salted, seasoned or not baked. Just stay away from anything laden with black list stuff.

TUNA (AND TINNED FISH) - Tinned fish is naturally going to contain levels of trace metals that you probably shouldn't be eating, so wherever possible – try for a non-tinned alternative. A lot of producers make tunas, etc. in plastic/foil wrapped packaging these days. As for the product itself, only ever go for the spring water option. Fish that is prepared in brine has a high salt content, which lends itself to the flavor of the product; and anything soaked in oil is completely unnecessary too. Always purchase from a leading brand, both for taste and quality, as you will quickly find out that a cheap tin of fish tastes like one. And that's no fun.

DAIRY – That means milk, cheese, yoghurts, ice cream - the lot. Always opt for a low fat or semi-skimmed option. Animal fats are big-ticket black list items and aren't great for anything to do with your sexual fitness. Don't go for anything complicated and processed in the dessert isle – goes without saying that it's going to be laden with sugars, artificial sweeteners and fats, and you can do a lot better yourself at home with real and better-for-you ingredients. Opt for a low-fat, organic frozen yoghurt over ice-creams (the latter as with most of the dessert isle will offer little nutritional value, whereas the frozen yoghurt will at least be naturally sweetened by a high fruit content and natural sugars and/or honey, vanilla bean, etc. Fresh milk is far better in the nutritional content you need and want to be getting out of it than anything UHT (long life), which although offers convenience has basically been nuked to allow it to sit in a carton for a questionably indefinite period of time. Not good and unnecessary. If you haven't tried organic, natural yoghurts that are set in a clay pot, you must. They taste great and contain little nasties other than some sugars, so try to go with the natural, unsweetened sort and sweeten yourself as needed, using honey or agave with a dash of Ceylon cinnamon or berries. So the best things you can possibly do as far as yoghurts are concerned are stick to natural yoghurts and low fat Greek yoghurt, which offers high levels of protein and basically all of the good stuff your body needs that's found in dairy products

FRUIT AND VEGETABLES – FRESH vs. TINNED vs. DRIED – You have eaten enough fresh fruit and vegetables during your detox to know that fresh is best and should always be your first preference. Tinned fruits are a little hit and miss. Despite the obvious fact that they contain trace metals and have been heat-treated, much like UHT milk, they also contain sugars, which really don't need to be there. It's not an unwise choice to keep away from tinned fruits as much as possible. Dried fruits are another of the world's great ambiguities. A candied fruit represents the equivalent of a bag of sugar, so you may as well be eating a bag of lollies – or better yet, not at all. You need to bear in mind that dried fruits are preserved using all those artificials that we're starting to love to hate, hence the reason a well and truly *dead* piece of fruit can somehow retain its original lustrous qualities. So scrap that – you will know a natural and organic dried apricot from the fact that it will be brown in color, and actually resemble that of a piece of fruit that's been dried in the sun. The labels *shouldn't* lie, so look for fruits that look naturally dried and always remember to check the label to make sure there's nothing unnecessary in there. Always be weary of labels and if in doubt, just forget about it and move on.

CARBS - RICES, PASTAS AND CEREALS – Carbs, carbs, carbs. One of the great temptations the world has to offer – and for good reason, they are a feel good food (add some of our favorite black list fat and sugar to the mix and you suddenly have yourself a doughnut – feeling *good* yet?). But let's keep them in check, just like everything else we're eating. Always go for the brown, natural option of which there's a lot to choose from now that the world has apparently turned healthy (which makes you wonder long and hard how contrasting the shades of black and white are, when you compare the organic, health food isle to the chips and sweets isle running down the other side). Cereals follow as much or a rule of thumb as our week's worth of general logic would suggest – nothing colored, sweetened, 'too good not to buy' kind of stuff. Try the natural, toasted mueslis, oats, bran, anything nut/flax – blue list type of thing. Honey sweetened and dark cocoa flavored organic cereal products are usually floating around somewhere. You will notice the package will be smaller and probably carry a slightly higher price tag, but keep two things in mind – the smaller packaging will usually resemble the *actual* contents of the product, opting for a more ecological packaging over a double bag/box situation - which as you know is usually like 50 something percent full *if that*. Secondly, a higher priced, higher quality product will have less commercial viability than the mass-produced, mass-appeal, value for money type low-cost general consumerism *shit*. We've been over that enough to know that it's not worth splitting hairs over adding a few cents more to a bowl of cereal. Your body says thank-you in advance!

HERBS & SPICES – Wherever possible, fresh is best. You can't beat the taste of fresh herbs and the ones that can live in your kitchen for easy daily use, should. Spices – only use organic from a quality, natural brand/supplier. These will represent a higher grade of product with little/no additives. Remember that few cents extra per serve thing? It very much applies here too. *Cheap* alternatives as you know can contain harmful byproducts. So as for that nutshell again: tasteless and pointless… You're better off donating that money to your local charity.

CHEAT-TREAT MEALS

Particularly in the first couple of days of your detox, you will have appreciated what 'cheat-treats' have been all about. The same is going to apply to your life going forward with your diet. Typically the life of an active and fit-conscious individual will involve 6 and half days of disciplined eating each week, followed by an evening out, *letting their hair down*. I'm no exception and nor should you be. We are all human – and the effectiveness of any balance that you achieve between red lists and yellow lists and blue lists and green lists will only be as effective as your own ability to keep a level head. And doing that means *just that* - rewarding yourself for a week's worth of structure, motivation and disciplined eating and lifestyle habits, by taking a night off and enjoying a guilt-free meal. Now that's going to mean something different for each of us, but as I've found, over the course of my journey with food – as you spend more time in the kitchen, playing around with ways to make the basic daily churn offer a level of continuous intrigue and appeal, you begin to develop tricks and techniques that make the most out of a food that you actually want to be eating. Be that completely natural teas, out of fruit and veg, (which you can easily become addicted to) or protein rich and carb-friendly desserts, made from stuff that's actually good for you and sweetened naturally, through to the daily grind of main meals that use great tasting fresh produce, allowing the simplicity of the quality ingredients to be the star of the show – I've come to love food. Notwithstanding the difference between a restaurant quality dessert for example and the one I will make at home according to my balance of lists, the difference is such that when I do go out and have my night off and enjoy something prepared by a pastry chef at one of my favorite restaurants – who will of course hold nothing back – it will be good enough to knock my socks off. And that's exactly what you want to achieve out of your *cheat-treat* – is that little personal indulgence that will reward the hell out of you and motivate you to get back on the horse the next morning, get active, stay disciplined and remember exactly why you signed onto this seven days in the first place.

THE REAL TRUTH ABOUT ALCOHOL..

'Hard liquors' are the spirits that are heavily chemically processed and long story short, aren't going to do your sexual fitness any favors - health and taste alike. Alcohol, much like coffee is one of those parts of your diet that you're likely not going to avoid entirely - and for good reason too. There's a string of various social and psychological benefits of *'moderated'* alcohol consumption (and well, yep there's times when not so *moderated* consumption is just plain needed, or *plain fun*). By this stage of your detox you're going to have put a fair amount of effort into your sexual fitness though, so chances are that you're not going to be too readily willing to throw that out the window *just yet*. As much as balance is one of the golden rules you will have learnt over the course of the past six days, you will be pleased to know that the 'red list' alcohol alternative to your 'black list' hard liquors is in a nutshell, not going to put all your hard work to waste. Not only is alcohol going to decrease the appeal of your sexual scent by a long shot, there are studies that have suggested it decreases the amount of testosterone in your blood — which is a bit of a downer, considering all the hard work we've been doing to achieve the exact opposite. Naturally fermented beers, which contain dramatically fewer chemicals (and lower amounts of alcohol) are generally not pasteurized (sake can be added to this list too) and that's something worth considering. Your body's biggest issue with processing preservatives, chemicals and non-organic food sources is the fact that the process of clearing these toxins out of your body will involve negative effects on both the physical state and most importantly your sexual scent. So as a general rule - be it applied towards alcohol, or any parts of your diet involving processed *crap* that falls into the above categories, the more natural you can set out to be with what goes in, the more organic will be the process of what you are getting out of your body - covering your sexual fitness as a whole. It's another one of those small things you can do, which will add up to the total sum of your efforts and in the long run help you achieve the best level of sexual health and fitness you can hope for.

So next time you're thinking of reaching for the whiskey and cola bottles - try knocking back a couple of natural 'boutique' beers instead. Not only are they increasing in popularity, they actually have very crisp and pure tasting notes attached to them, and are available in a considerable varsity of brews - dark, light and even honey (for non-beer drinkers looking to avoid that *beer* taste at all costs), so you're bound to find one that you will take a liking to. And honestly speaking - after you have sampled a good selection of these boutique natural beers and appreciate the simple complexities in the quality of taste they offer, you're going to be hard pressed to reach for any old bottle of beer again after that.

SUGGESTED WARM SPICED BEER RECIPE

Warm spiced beer is largely popular in Europe, particularly during the cooler (winter) months (which is basically most of the year!) It's easy to throw together and involves basically heating your favorite natural, unpasteurized beer on a low heat, without boiling – whilst stirring through your own spice mix, which ultimately makes it a blue list/red list *acceptable* beverage. Adding honey (less or more depending on how sweet you're into) enhances this drink less the need for sugar.

Make up your own spice mix by combining: Ceylon cinnamon, cloves, + nutmeg with any of the following that you're into: cardamom, allspice, star anise (natural and ground of course - quality natural suppliers should have powdered options available). As a general guide, 2 parts cinnamon (as a base) to 1 part of anything else will give you a well-rounded spice mix. ½-1 teaspoon to a bottle of beer should be enough to spice your beer nicely.

SUGGESTED COCKTAIL - SAKE SEX DRIVE

Mix.
0.5L cold green tea + 0.5L freshly squeezed pomegranate juice + 4 shots natural sake + juice of half a lemon.
Stir.
Serve on ice.

DAY SEVEN – 'GREAT SEX DAY'

Go for gold - and always taste like it too

Tonight's the big night when you and your playmate get to start over, and as far as first dates go – this ones going to have a very happy ending ☺

EXPECTED ENERGY-MENTAL ALERTNESS-HUNGER LEVELS FOR DAY SEVEN

Energy –
Morning: ***high***
Afternoon: ***high***
Evening: ***high then low***

Mental Alertness –
Morning: ***high***
Afternoon: ***high***
Evening: ***high then low***

Hunger –
Morning: ***high then low***
Afternoon: ***high then low***
Evening: ***high then low***

Day seven of your detox is based on three main goals:
One – *LIFESTYLE MAINTENANCE PHASE*
Two – *SEXUAL FITNESS MAINTENANCE PHASE*
Three – *NUTRITIONAL PLANNING CHALLENGE*

1. 'LIFESTYLE MAINTENANCE' PHASE - In summary – it's time to apply all the lifestyle choices you know are good for your sexual fitness and put them to permanent use. Understanding some of the basics in daily meal preparation, whilst working with the foods you will consume on a typical day is going to make all the difference. Also knowing how to cut the right corners to avoid making mistakes *in bad taste,* without falling into the pit of boredom too easily is going to help you a lot. Spare a thought to those of us who have various food allergies or for example, lactose intolerance – they still manage to get by somehow, right? So all you really need to do is think of your black list as a list of these intolerances your body can't and shouldn't have to worry about, and soon enough you will realize that you can in fact live without them, and yep – manage to *get by.*

2. 'SEXUAL FITNESS MAINTENANCE' PHASE - It's all about making newly formed good habits stay that way, so keep things in perspective by checking up on what you're doing going forward and being on the front foot with any changes you need to make, as you need to make them. Your playmate is going to be an important check on your sexual fitness – so use them to make sure everything's going according to plan. Remember back to some of that open and honest communication we discovered doesn't happen as often as it should back on day one – well today's the day when you can change all that (and as a matter of fact the success of the outcome of your detox could be attributed to it) by learning to pop the big question, *'so, did it taste alright?'* If your detox has gone according to plan, a happy set of lips should be all the recognition you need for your hard work over the past seven days. Whereas if you're running solo, you should yourself be able to self-evaluate the success of your week by taking a look at the small things that have changed for the better. And perhaps it's time to start looking for a new playmate? ☺

3. NUTRITIONAL PLANNING CHALLENGE – Over the course of the past six days you've developed a sense of what's going to contribute positively to your sexual fitness and what's going to get in the way of your sexual scent. Today's challenge is to plan ahead for the coming week, so you can transfer your newfound good habits into user-friendly daily meal plans that will help form a positive set of ongoing eating habits.

You're going to need paper and pen and your overall goal is to create a daily run sheet for the following seven, broken down into your three main meals and three snacks, much like the general pattern you have been following throughout your detox. Entering into an organized phase of eating regular meals is going to be much simpler everyday, when you have a visual guide that's going to be useful for both shopping and for knowing what you're eating at home and what's being packed to go, for when you're not at home. The Internet is going to be your best friend both for this challenge and going forward. There's an endless supply of recipes, ideas, inspiration that can be used to turn an otherwise basic meal into something both visually stimulating and palette-friendly. Remember the basics that you picked up on in the first couple of days of your detox, when you were eating less and were therefore far more receptive to enjoying the taste of simple things - such as adding fruit to a salad. By this stage you will have a feel for the simple ways that black listers can be replaced with better-for-you alternatives. And being more conscious of what blue listers for example can be added to complement or enhance an otherwise plain boring or plain unhealthy recipe will open up a world of food friendly variations to any old recipe you can find on the net. So on that note, use your red, green and yellow lists to create a good balanced diet, and don't forget to use your blue list to pack your meals full of the foods that will give your sexual fitness a great edge!

NUTRITIONAL PLANNING CHALLENGE

So to sum it up - for your nutritional planning challenge, use the following template to create a seven-day meal plan, and make use of the shopping list and quick recipe guide in the back of the book to help you out!

MONDAY MEALS *(or day one meals, etc.)*

BREAKFAST *(or meal 1 etc.)*Glass of water/fruit water/fruit tea +

SNACK Glass of water/fruit water/fruit tea +

LUNCH Glass of water/fruit water/fruit tea +

SNACK Glass of water/fruit water/fruit tea +

DINNER Glass of water/fruit water/fruit tea +

SNACK Glass of water/fruit water/fruit tea +

*And as far as 'glasses' are concerned, I dislike ambiguity – so pick up a new favorite glass that's about half a L in size and use that from now on (none of this sippy cup 200ML glass BS ☺)

DAY SEVEN MEAL PLAN

BREAKFAST
1+ L OF WATER (plus another 1+ L in-between meals)
Warm orange soup with Greek yoghurt and organic muesli
Whole-wheat toast with homemade jam
A cup of coffee/tea

SNACK
A LARGE GLASS OF WATERMELON + POMEGRANATE SMOOTHIE
(With yellow list mixed in)
2 tablespoons fresh peanut butter

LUNCH
1 + L OF WATER (plus another 1+ L in-between meals)
Whole-wheat sandwich stuffed with salad + chicken or tuna

SNACK
A LARGE GLASS OF WATERMELON + POMEGRANATE JUICE
(With yellow list mixed in)
Fresh fruits (keep that yellow list going)
2 hardboiled eggs

DINNER
1+ L OF WATER
Oven roasted turkey breast with steamed/roasted vegetables or a flat bread pizza
Baked apple

SNACK
Baked popcorn chicken nuggets

BAKED CINNAMON APPLE WITH HONEY RECIPE

This is a healthy and wholesome dessert - and even better served piping hot out of the oven, especially on a cold day. Throw a fireplace into the works, invite your playmate over for *dessert* and you're set for a really good night in.

1. Preheat a fan forced or convection oven to 220C/430F degrees

2. Core a large apple per person (the bigger the better) and stuff with some freshly grated orange peel, ginger, organic raisins, unsweetened and naturally ground Ceylon cinnamon powder. Also try adding some shaved nutmeg for an extra kick! Top with an organic honey and bake for 30 minutes, or until the apples have puffed out and the skin starts to come off.

3. Serve alongside some low fat Greek yoghurt lightly covered with some shaved orange peel and dark chocolate and a drizzle of honey.

FLATBREAD PIZZA RECIPE

This is by far the easiest and healthiest attempt at a pizza you're likely going to come into contact with, and it seriously takes like 10 minutes to throw together plus oven time, so preheat your oven to 180/350 degrees

1. Using a whole-wheat piece of flatbread, place on a baking tray and prepare a simple sauce out of Greek yoghurt and an organic tomato sauce (which should be sugar and nasty-free), apply generously

2. Add any amount of healthy toppings – roast pork, pan cooked ham, roast beef, capsicum, red onion, pineapple, mushrooms, cottage cheese and some low-fat grated cheese.

3. Bake for 15 minutes and after it's out of the oven, top with some fresh rucola. See? I wasn't kidding when I said it was both healthy and really taste bud-friendly!

POPCORN CHICKEN NUGGETS RECIPE

Another example of making healthy, user-friendly.

Pre-heat your oven to 180/350 degrees and slice a chicken breast into nugget size chunks. Dip in a beaten egg, before rolling around in some popcorn flour.

Bake for 15-20 minutes and yep, it's that easy.

How to go about making the popcorn flour? Also nothing to loose sleep over – throw a cup or two of popcorn into the food processor and mix on high for a couple of minutes, until you've achieved a completely flour-like powder. The result – a completely taste and fitness-friendly coating for a clean protein nugget that's black list free.

SIMPLE HOMEMADE JAM RECIPE

There's ways to enjoy some of those comfy foods you have grown up with, just like you have discovered with peanut butter. A simple homemade jam (less the three tablespoons of sugar that comes with each teaspoon) is no exception.

Take a generous serving of a naturally sweet fruit such as ripe raspberries, cherries, plums or nectarines, pit and reduce in a small saucepan on a slow boil. Add honey for added sweetness (1-2 tablespoons should do the trick) along with a few teaspoons of fresh lemon juice (which will help it set). Continue to heat for 10 minutes until you've achieved a thick fruit sauce and pour into a jar that you've sterilized with boiling water, and leave to set. After it's cooled it's fine to be refrigerated for a couple of days, which should give you about enough time to dish it up a couple of times for breakfast. If you're looking for something more jelly-jam like, don't forget about the agar you've used in your fruit jellies, to firm up your breakfast spread.

And what's more – scoffing a natural peanut butter and jam sandwich for late night snacks couldn't really get any better could it?

ALMOND LEMON BALLS RECIPE

Use these two recipes for snacks – they're packed with simple blue list friendly ingredients and are a great alternative to the usual black list snacks you're avoiding.

You will need:
- A cup of raw almonds
- Rind from a lemon
- A half cup of organic dried apricots or plums

1. Using your food processor, grind the almonds until they turn into powder form
2. Add the remaining ingredients until the mixture achieves a dough like consistency
3. Roll into balls (tablespoon size) and roll through desiccated coconut and refrigerate

CASHEW DATE SLICE RECIPE

You will need:
- A cup of raw cashews
- A cup of organic, unsweetened, pitted dates
- 1 teaspoon grated ginger

1. Using your food processor, grind the cashews until they turn into powder form
2. Add the remaining ingredients until the mixture achieves a slightly oily dough like consistency
3. Spread onto a shallow, baking paper lined baking tray and pack the mixture down firmly, before refrigerating

GENERAL NOTES ON
MEAL PREPARATION

Making simple changes to the way you do things can bring about good lifestyle changes. In the spirit of leaving your black list of foods well alone, use the following as a guide to alternative black list foods:

OVEN BAKE *instead of fry* – using a light coating and a healthy spray oil will give you a naturally golden finish and *virtually no fat*

GRILL *instead of pan fry* – using a good quality skillet at a moderate-high temp and a light spray of your preferred healthy oil if required, to produce a lightly crisped finish

LESS SALT *is more as far as your sexual fitness is concerned* – you can achieve similar flavor intensities with a minimal amount of salt, placing the focus on achieving a bold flavor with natural herbs and blue list foods. Try a sweet alternative, such as a fig, ginger and honey glazed chicken – over a honey soy combo for example. All the intensity *none of the salt* – or opt for a low sodium(salt) alternative

GREEN SALT *is a healthier choice* – look for a natural spirulina (or algae) sea salt in your health store (or on the internet). It's finely ground and contains spirulina, which is a superfood offering a massive amount of vitamins and minerals

DRESS UP *by dressing down* – using a simple lemon and good oil dressing for a salad is going to top any store bought vinaigrette any day. Crack some fresh pepper in with a pinch of salt and try adding some organic ginger powder and/or paprika if that's missing too

MAKE YOUR OWN *carbonated soft drink alternatives* – add equal parts natural mineral water to your favorite juice blend and try that for refreshment

NATURALLY SWEET *is always best* – use honey and agave nectars instead of sugars to sweeten whatever needs it

BROWN IS BEST *as far as sugar is concerned* – if you're going to run into the need to use sugar at some point down the track, which you inevitably will, use an unrefined, natural brown sugar, sparingly. Try an organic coconut sugar too as an alternative.

SPICE IT DOWN *by using your blue list herbs and spices to replace the strong black listers* – coriander/lemongrass/ginger will kick chilly's ass any day

CRAVING CAULIFLOWER? Take an extra meal out of your cheat day and go nuts. Even cover it in a nice white sauce. Just remember that's going to cost you an extra L of water and a glass of fresh orange juice for dessert!

GREASE IT UP *without using very much at all* – Healthy oils such as rice bran, olive oil, avocado oil, flax oil, walnut oil used in a spray bottle will lightly cover whatever needs covering and keep it light. Plain and simple

What does "organic" mean anyway? It's a term that's been used throughout this book to mean natural and unprocessed in the case of store bought produce, including fresh and packaged. It's referring to a choice of product that contains none of the black listers we have been learning to avoid and basically a smart alternative to commercial and processed foods that offer little nutritional value.

MICROWAVES – despite convenience, offer little else to the nutritional value of your finished product. Nuke for 30 sec, and you may as well be eating a powdered mash out of a box. Still interested?

TUPPERWARE AND ZIPLOCS – can be your friend with leftover meals and fruit and vegetables that are going straight for the juicer tomorrow. It keeps everything fresh and reduces wastage.

SCRUB AWAY AT
ALL THAT BAD

You will have been busy dry brushing for the past week, so now it's time to step it up a notch and make for some seriously tasty scrubbing, which will make your body feel great and prep you for that big night in with your playmate. Natural at-home body scrubs are really simple to make, you guessed it — out of some of the same wholesome ingredients that you have been feeding your body with for the past seven days. You're treating your body to a super stimulating all-over polish, so going to town with a little bit of sugar is actually going to be great for this exercise! Try one of these few recipes on for size and remember to light some candles, get that *Lana del Ray* thing going on and scrub out every last bit of bad that should no longer be there, like the rest of your night depends on it!

While you're down there — have you taken to all and everything with a pair of clippers recently? You will find that most playmates will appreciate a well-groomed (clean) workspace any day of the week. For those of us guys that haven't considered it before — it's actually nowhere near as unfriendly as you may have made it out to be. We're not talking shaving/waxing/any majorly intrusive procedures here — what you should be using is a basic "body groomer" (clipper). They're available everywhere, shouldn't set you back more than your yoga mat for a halfway decent one and are basically an extended, *body hair* version of your good old electric razor. So no nicks, cuts, pain, ingrown hairs, or angst really. It's easy to DIY — but you can always get your playmate to *lend you a helping hand.* ☺

COOKIE DOUGH SCRUB

You will need:
- 1-cup organic brown sugar
- ¼ cup coconut oil (unrefined)
- 1-teaspoon cinnamon (or more if you like)
- ½ teaspoon pure vanilla essential oil (that's about 20 drops)

If the coconut oil is solid (in temperatures below 24/76 degrees) then warm over a low heat to soften, before adding to a small bowl and whisking through the brown sugar and cinnamon. Mix will (so there's no lumps) before adding the vanilla and giving it one more go. Massage well into the body, dampening the skin a little if you need to (damp skin will make for a more thorough scrub). The result? You should be smelling, tasting, feeling something along the lines of cookie dough by now – so don't go acting too surprised if your playmate doesn't even let you out of the bathroom. I guess showering together *can* save water *whilst* helping you to get at all those…*hard to reach* places.

BUTTER UP

You've scrubbed up quite well it seems – the last seven days look to have done you a world of good. Now finish up by covering yourself from head to toe in a deliciously whipped natural cocoa butter, so you can taste every bit as good on the outside as you will be on the inside. And it seems like our job here is just about done – the rest of night seven all depends on you. Your playmate awaits - and the rest? Well let's just say that we both know what part of the bitter-sweet sex story you're going to be all about.

THE FINAL WORD

IT'S FAIRLY ACCURATE to think of your overall sexual fitness and particularly your sexual scent as being the most easily recognizable element of a blueprint for overall health and balance of what you do with your body. When it comes to having a great sex life, every last bit of what you put into your body will determine everything that you get out of it, when you need it the most. And what you do get out of your body - especially when your playmate's watching, is going to let them know exactly how committed you are to your sexual relationship. *A committed* playmate is a *happy* playmate, and a happy playmate is a *satisfied* and *great tasting* one. You're satisfied because B is impressed and willing to do things that only last week it seems, were so far from being great - no one was really having that much fun. And we all no that no fun in the bedroom pretty much sucks. So now that you've discovered how to go about turning things around, you will be keen to explore that the best way to enjoy your sexuality is when there's nothing holding *you* or *your playmate* back. Part of this successful relationship with your playmate that you've been working hard to build on in this past week means even stepping things up a notch and knocking over this detox together. Once you're in the swing of things, doing it twice a year to keep everything fresh (every six months, let's say – particularly after the 'wet' summer *drinking* months) isn't necessarily the worst idea to be had for keeping your sexual fitness at its peak.

Think of your sexual fitness as a long term investment – the more you chip away at it, the greater the chance it will keep working for you for longer than you've likely even contemplated needing it. And even if you're not using it – it's one of those personal positive attributes that you can never have enough of. Your sexual fitness is going to speak louder than words in your overall level of personal *pull power*, self-satisfaction and most importantly – self esteem. And if in the least we can take one of those honest *long, hard look in the mirror* moments and feel good about ourselves, then truth be told - we're doing all right.

And it's a sure thing that someone else will see that too.

So eating healthy, living well - what does it all have to do with your sexual fitness anyway? Short answer – pretty much everything you've managed to pick up on over the course of the past seven days.

Still hate cum as much as you did this time last week? I didn't think so.